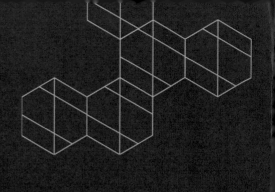

BLOOD SUGAR
DOESN'T LIE

How Hidden Blood Sugar Imbalance Drives
Chronic Disease and Brain Disorders –
and Your Guide to Fixing It!

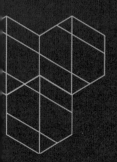

WELL CENTERS

f8wellcenters.com

Written by

Dr. Ben Galyardt

F8 Well Centers

Published and Designed
by Meazzo Design Co.

A NOTE FROM DR. BEN

Blood sugar is a term that gets thrown around alot in the world of diabetes and obesity and yet many people overlook how glucose fluctuation can contribute to most chronic disease states. After 20 plus years in practice I have come to the conclusion that over 90% of chronic conditions could be reversed or prevented if we did one simple thing: Stabilize everyone's blood glucose levels between 85-110. This may be simple, but not always easy. In this book I am going to show you the process we go through with patients in order to figure out which foods make their glucose levels rise and why they crash down at other times. You will also learn the damaging effects not only high glucose causes in the body but also lows and especially the extreme swings from high to low and back again. This is truly the foundational piece we have found while working with thousands of patients from around the world - glucose stability.

The body is a complex organism where systems can get out of balance and cause a cascade effect down the chain. We try to maintain homeostasis and not get too revved up or too depleted, but like goldilocks - just right. We have seen so many lives changed by getting a patient's blood sugar stabilized that this has to be the place to start for you. Whether you are starting from a place of diabetes, autoimmune, weight gain, brain issues or countless other issues, begin with blood sugar as your foundational piece and you will see miracles take place in your health.

To Your Wellness:

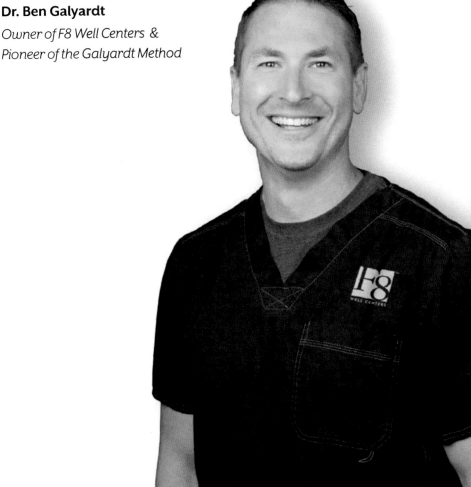

Dr. Ben Galyardt
Owner of F8 Well Centers &
Pioneer of the Galyardt Method

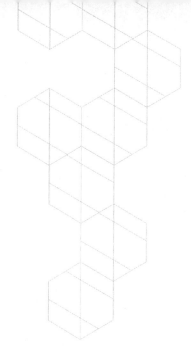

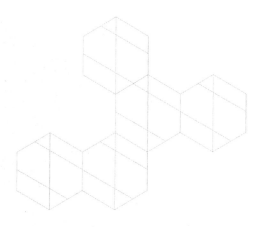

TABLE OF CONTENTS

CHAPTER 1

The New Blood **Sugar Paradigm**

SARAH'S STORY

When I first examined Sarah, a 40-year-old mother of three young kids, her symptoms didn't align with the healthy-looking person I saw in front of me. Just moments into her neurological exam, it was clear that looks can be deceiving.

"Do you have a history of stroke?" I asked.

I was not being flippant - her neurological signs were concerning. She struggled to walk a straight line or complete a coherent sentence. Sarah was not your average patient; she was very attuned to her health. She was not only a meditation teacher but also lived on a small farm, growing vegetables and raising her chickens and children. Her diet was based on whole and organic foods, and she exercised regularly. However, something was "off" deep within her cells, leading to dangerous and terrifying symptoms, and we needed to figure out what it was.

While Sarah's laboratory results didn't indicate a blood sugar imbalance, I suspected we weren't seeing the whole picture. In fact, her HbA1c, which measures average blood sugar over three months, was perfect at 5.0. Although, when I sent her home with a glucometer to track her blood sugar before and after meals, we saw a very different story.

Sarah was waking up with very low blood glucose levels of 70 but spiking up to 200 after eating ½ an apple. She uncovered other strange foods that were raising her blood sugar levels too high like broccoli, sauerkraut, carrots and matcha tea. This made her average blood glucose look great, but in reality, she was on a blood sugar roller coaster from morning 'til night.

Through a conventional medical lens, these symptoms are impossibly hard to believe. For me, this has become the norm. My patients come in with symptoms ranging from cancer to multiple sclerosis, chronic fatigue to attention deficit. Often, they arrive with no diagnosis but a general feeling of failing health. Each time, we find a unique blood sugar pattern that gives us an indisputable look into how their bodies are reacting to the foods they eat.

Most healthcare professionals would tell you that your blood sugar will rise in a direct response to the amount of carbs you eat. For instance, if you eat a slice of white bread or drink a soda, we would expect your blood sugar to increase more than if you eat the same amount of carbohydrates in a sweet potato or a bowl of brown rice. Generally, this may be true for someone who is very healthy. However, our patients' glucose responses paint a very different picture.

Over the course of health degradation, they have often lost the ability to metabolize carbohydrates properly or they've developed extreme responses to specific foods. This leads to whacky and individualized blood sugar spikes and dips, often totally unrelated to the level of carbohydrates they've recently consumed.

Linda is an example. She was diagnosed with multiple sclerosis over 15 years ago and had it well controlled until a devastating breast cancer diagnosis led to chemotherapy in 2015. While chemo killed the cancer, it left her unable to function physically and mentally. Her neurological system took a huge hit, and the lesions in her brain grew.

When Linda and I began working together, it was her "Hail Mary." Nothing else had worked, and she had been forced to quit her job and dig into her savings to pay her medical bills and survive. Her primary care doctor told her that her symptoms were irreversible and that it was time to begin utilizing harsh drugs to treat her progressive MS.

We got to work investigating Linda's unique cellular function. While we waited for laboratory diagnostics to come in, she began testing her blood sugar throughout the day. While sugary foods and wine were spiking her blood sugar, she also identified consistent blood sugar spikes after eating chicken, tomatoes, eggplant, peppers and potatoes.

Linda was also dealing with neuropathy as a side effect from the cancer drug Tamoxifen, so we began supporting her healing with neurofeedback and other helpful therapies such as pulsed electromagnetic field therapy. In the meantime, she removed all of the foods that caused her blood sugar to stray from healthy ranges. Within two weeks, she began to report feeling like she was "waking up." The fog in her brain was lifting, and she was getting sensation back in her fingers.

Around three months into treatment, Linda felt like her old self, better than she did prior to her cancer. She is currently awaiting her annual brain scan and is expecting to see that her lesions have improved. She says that if how she feels is any indication, they may be gone. Linda experiments by incorporating some of the foods we eliminated from her diet, but each time she does, she begins to feel the symptoms she worked so hard to get rid of. At this point, she's happy to live without chicken, wine and nightshade vegetables if it means feeling "alive" each and every day.

In an interesting contrast, another patient who has dealt with a frustrating autoimmune condition for almost a decade found that a glass of red wine keeps her blood sugar in optimal ranges; however, almond milk sends her blood sugar through the roof. For her, intermittent fasting and any level of calorie restriction causes imbalanced blood sugar, even though those practices can be helpful for others. This illustrates how individualized blood sugar responses can be.

Why Does Imbalanced Blood Sugar Cause So Many Problems?

The body works very hard to keep its many systems in balance, and all of those systems are interconnected. This means that when your blood sugar is out of balance, the body has to call on other systems to help it balance your blood sugar. For instance, if your blood sugar is too low (which is extremely dangerous), the body reacts with a stress response. That triggers the adrenal glands to release the stress hormone cortisol. Cortisol then triggers the liver to release stored glucose into the bloodstream to bring blood sugar back into a healthy range.

However, this raises cortisol in the body, which eventually leads to inflammation and a domino effect of other health problems.

The same can be said for high blood sugar. Sugar is supposed to travel into cells where it can be used as energy. When there's too much sugar in the bloodstream, it requires more and more insulin to help it enter the cells. Excess insulin is also inflammatory, which results in tissue damage throughout the body. While your back pain, brain fog or autoimmune condition may seem unrelated, it's the inflammatory response from imbalanced blood sugar that links them together. Imagine that this dysregulation occurs beneath the surface every day for months or years. At some point, the body will have had enough and won't be able to fight off a full-blown disease.

But I'm getting ahead of myself. Before I dive into the link between blood sugar and the chronic disease epidemic that is plaguing our country (and my patients), let's take a few steps back and make sure we're all up to speed on how food becomes fuel. While you read through the next section, don't get overwhelmed by details. Instead, focus on the big picture, the importance of a well-functioning digestive system. Later, we'll use this information to better understand how to create a diet that stabilizes your blood sugar and energy all day. Let's dive in.

NOTES

CHAPTER 2

How Food
Becomes Fuel

MARIE'S STORY

Marie was 39 years old when we began working together. She was 150 pounds overweight with an HbA1c over 6.0, in spite of taking Metformin daily. Regardless of the many hours she was spending at the gym each week, her weight was creeping up and her energy was low.

Worse than the uncontrolled blood sugar and spiraling weight gain was her growing loss of interest in life. Marie felt angry and depressed all the time. She had pulled away from family and was avoiding social events.

We got to work identifying foods that were spiking her blood sugar while we supported her gut and liver function. Quickly, weight began to melt away and before long, her HbA1c was under 5.7 without medication. Within 9 months, she had lost over 75 pounds and she felt engaged in life again.

Her depression was gone, and she felt energized and happy. Notably excited to spend time with her nephews and nieces again, her family told her that they felt like she had "come back to them".

For most of us, we normally think of sweets when we talk about eating sugar, but everything from fruit to corn chips and beans contains sugar. Sugars are the tiny molecules that form carbohydrates. When carbohydrates are broken down through digestion, they eventually become the disaccharides (2-sugar molecules). Maltose, lactose or sucrose are then further broken down into fructose, glucose and galactose, which are referred to as monosaccharides or 1-sugar molecules.

The end result of all carbohydrates whether they're stored in fruits, vegetables, legumes, bread, pasta, dairy, rice, corn or desserts. Every time you eat a carbohydrate, the end-product-monosaccharide is absorbed into the bloodstream, which increases the level of sugar in the blood. While eating too many carbohydrates—especially refined sources like candy, cookies, chips or white bread— can raise pretty much anyone's blood sugar to excessive levels, all carbohydrates aren't bad.

In fact, carbohydrates are our primary fuel source for the body and brain. Carbohydrates can provide a quick energy boost because they're more easily digested and absorbed into the bloodstream compared to fats, our other major fuel source. Our bodies innately know how to turn food into fuel and other building blocks that our bodies need to function, but it is far from a simple process. Even small malfunctions in the chain of events between chewing and food absorption can derail this process and lead to a host of health problems.

Turning Food into Fuel and Function

For food to break down into the tiny components that can be absorbed into circulation, robust digestive function is required. Once the microscopic molecules are absorbed, they're used to generate energy and support every biochemical process the body needs to operate. While this is quite a complex process, it's important to have a basic understanding of how this works before diving into a deeper conversation about blood sugar.

Imagine that you just ate a stereotypical American breakfast consisting of eggs and potatoes. Potatoes contain carbohydrates (primarily starch and fiber) and water, while eggs are rich in protein and fats. These foods also contain micronutrients such as vitamins, minerals and other healthy phytochemicals. Carbohydrates, proteins and fats are "large" molecules (macronutrients) and must be broken down to their small components before they are absorbed. There are small proteins called enzymes throughout the digestive tract (mouth to colon) that aid in the disassembly of large molecules to their small components.

Let's follow your breakfast. Digestion begins in the mouth as soon as you begin to chew. Although many people rush through this part of digestion, chewing is really important. Chewing not only breaks down food into smaller pieces, making it easier to digest, but also integrates the food with saliva at this time. Saliva contains amylase and lipase, enzymes that help disassemble carbohydrates and fats, respectively. Have you ever been told that you should chew each bite 30 times? This is why.

Now your pasty bite of eggs and potato can be swallowed down your esophagus and into your stomach. Your mushy bite has arrived in your stomach, the primary site of protein digestion. Thanks to this fist-sized organ situated under the sternum, your protein-rich eggs are about to be unraveled and taken apart. When your stomach senses food, it secretes a critical fluid called gastric juice, a mixture of protective mucous, hydrochloric acid (HCl), intrinsic factor, and digestive enzymes.

Each component has an important and specialized job: HCl (stomach acid) unravels proteins, releasing micronutrients such as vitamin B-12 and iron from tightly bound protein molecules, while mucous coats and protects the stomach cells from the acid. Stomach acid has the dual benefit of killing dangerous microbes like bacteria within your food. Intrinsic factor is not involved in digestion but is necessary for transporting the essential vitamin B-12 into the intestines so that it can be absorbed.

HCl also stimulates stomach enzymes that help to continue protein digestion and begin fat break down. Lastly, the stomach secretes a hormone called gastrin. Gastrin signals the pancreas that food is on its way so that it can release pancreatic digestive enzymes while the gallbladder secretes bile (a fat emulsifier).

Now your breakfast has morphed into chyme, a mushy mixture of gastric juices and partially digested food bits, and is ready for the final processes of digestion. As your breakfast leaves the stomach en route to the intestines, the acidic mixture from the stomach needs to be neutralized so that your delicate intestinal cells aren't damaged.

A helpful hormone called secretin signals the pancreas to produce an alkaline bicarbonate fluid while also triggering the stomach to stop producing gastrin. This is a great example of the innate wisdom of internal communication systems. So, it makes sense that when these intricate communication processes get off track, they become vulnerable to disease. Imagine that secretin was not produced in enough quantity to produce bicarb, therefore neutralizing stomach acid. Your intestinal cells would become susceptible to damage and could no longer absorb food efficiently.

But secretin is just getting started. Its next role is to tell the pancreas to secrete a blend of digestive enzymes and notify the gallbladder to release bile. Pancreatic juices work to further break down proteins into amino acids, lipids into smaller fatty acids and carbohydrates such as starch and sugar into disaccharides. Fiber, on the other hand, won't be digested but will continue its journey to the colon.

By now, your breakfast is unrecognizable, primed for the last steps before nutrients can be absorbed into circulation. The brush border (surface of your intestinal cells) house brush border enzymes, which are ready to perform the final task of breaking amino acids down and transforming carbohydrates from disaccharides (2-sugar molecules of lactose, sucrose and maltose) into monosaccharides (1-sugar molecules of glucose, galactose and fructose).

Some people, due to genetics or intestinal damage, don't produce enough brush border enzymes to complete this phase of digestion efficiently. Lactose-intolerance is a great example and a common condition that occurs when people don't produce enough of the lactase enzyme to break lactose into glucose and galactose. This means that lactose isn't digested or absorbed well, resulting in nasty digestive symptoms like bloating, diarrhea or constipation.

While most food bits are now absorbed into circulation, some particles will travel with fiber into the colon. Fiber from vegetables, fruits, grains, nuts, seeds and legumes is crucial to maintaining good health, reducing risk of common chronic diseases like colon cancer, diabetes, cardiovascular disease and obesity.[1] Fiber slows down the digestive process, which reduces the speed of sugar absorption into the blood, maintaining better blood sugar regulation. It also helps remove toxins and waste from the body.

There are two types of fiber: soluble and insoluble. Soluble fiber found in foods like flax, barley, psyllium, carrots, citrus, apples and oats helps lower cholesterol and glucose levels. Insoluble fiber like nuts, beans and vegetables bulk up your stool and move food and waste through the digestive process.

Fiber Feeds Your Healthy Gut Bacteria

Fiber boosts your health and consuming a variety of fiber plays an important role in feeding the microbiota in the colon. Technically, humans don't digest fiber, but small bacteria and other microbes in the colon (your microbiome) use many of the fibers you consume for their own fuel.

Building and maintaining a diverse and healthy microbiome decreases the volume of dangerous microbes that promote disease. Specific fermentable fibers (prebiotics) such as inulin, galacto-oligosaccharides (GOS) and fructo-oligosaccharides (FOS) feed your good "bugs," increase the number of colonies of healthy bacteria within the colon while improving gut barrier function, and balance the immune system.[2] Additionally, having healthy microbiota increases the production of short-chain fatty acids, which boost the immune system, protect the colon, improve metabolism, and enhance central nervous system function.[3,4] You also need a robust gut microbiome for the production and regulation of neurotransmitters and hormones, which support mental health.[4] A high-fiber diet does wonders for blood sugar control, helping to slow digestion and, therefore, regulate blood sugar. An added bonus is that fiber supports a healthy microbiome.

A Quick Time Out

Before moving on, let me just underscore the incredible importance of a highly functioning digestive system. If any of these processes don't occur appropriately, you'll suffer digestive problems, and your diet will lose its power to nourish and fuel you. If you're eating a standard American diet, then processed food, alone, can destroy the digestion process. That not only means your diet is lacking nutrients but also that your body will struggle to digest the nutrition you are getting.

Moving Nutrients into You

Up until this point, your digested food is actually still considered to be outside of you. Food is not part of you until the nutrients are absorbed across the intestinal barrier and into your circulation. Now that your breakfast is a "soup" of monosaccharides, amino acids, fatty acids and micronutrients, these small molecules must move into your bloodstream. Particles are absorbed through (not between) the intestinal cells and then sent out the other side into the bloodstream.

How Absorption Raises Blood Sugar

Are you asking yourself what all of this has to do with blood sugar? When glucose, the main monosaccharide, moves through the intestinal cells into circulation, the amount of sugar in the blood rises temporarily. This is a normal state and doesn't cause a problem if your body can effectively move glucose from the blood into the cells where it can be turned into energy. It's when the body loses this function that things go awry.

If things are moving along well, then once sugar enters your circulation, the pancreas secretes insulin. This is critical because insulin is required for glucose to be taken in by cells. If this function is totally shut down, you would have to take insulin injections to regulate blood sugar.

In essence, insulin is the chaperone to glucose. Insulin arrives with glucose at the cell and gives the cell's doorbell a ring saying "Yoo-hoo, we're here." Then, from deep within the center of the cells, a "glucose-greeter" floats up to the cell's surface to gather and accompany glucose inside. Once glucose enters the cell, insulin detaches from the cell's surface and returns to the liver to be recycled.

Problems with Blood Sugar

Now that we've covered how carbohydrates are broken down, absorbed and transported into cells, we can talk about how this process can go haywire. Consider a few possibilities that might go wrong and affect the amount of glucose within the bloodstream. For instance, what if a gush of glucose enters the blood, and the pancreas cannot produce enough insulin to accompany all the glucose into cells? What if the insulin docks on the cell, but the cell ignores it and doesn't send a greeter? What if the pancreas responds to a delivery of glucose in the bloodstream by delivering too much insulin, and there's not enough glucose left in the blood leading to low blood sugar?

To complicate matters even more, as I mentioned earlier, cortisol can cause stored glucose to be released into the bloodstream too regularly. Or, what if other hormones are interfering with insulin? The list is endless! If this process is not regulated, you may be ping-ponging back and forth between low and high blood sugar without ever knowing it.

Hypoglycemia

"Hypo" means under, so hypoglycemia means that blood sugar levels are low. This can happen if you wait too long to eat and your body doesn't have enough circulating sugar to fuel the surrounding cells, leaving them starved for energy. This may also happen because your body is producing too much insulin, or the meal you ate last was digested too quickly.

You may feel symptoms like fatigue, low energy, brain fog and may even pass out. You've probably heard the term "Hangry" to describe these symptoms, combining hungry and angry! In extreme low blood sugar situations, if the body runs out of ways to compensate, a person will die.

Skipping a meal is not usually cause for concern because the body has a few backup systems. One of those backup plans is cortisol, produced by the adrenal glands. As we already covered, cortisol stimulates the muscle and liver storage cells to release stored glucose back into the bloodstream.

This is because liver and muscle cells can store glucose as glycogen, a branched chain of a lot of glucose that resembles a tree. When blood sugar levels drop, cortisol tells those cells to disassemble and release sugar into the blood. This is why we say that the number one stressor to the adrenals is extreme blood sugar fluctuation. If one's blood sugar is continually spiking and dropping, the adrenal glands are under pressure trying to compensate with enough cortisol.

Hypoglycemia can also occur when too much insulin is present, as I mentioned earlier. If the pancreas releases too much insulin after glucose is absorbed into the blood, glucose may be taken up into cells too quickly, and your blood sugar drops too low. This is a big concern for many individuals suffering from either type 1 or type 2 diabetes who are taking insulin to manage their blood sugar. In these cases, if a person takes too much insulin in relation to the amount of glucose consumed, they will experience hypoglycemia and will need to quickly eat or drink carbohydrates to bring their blood sugar back up. Some people who do not have any form of diabetes but who may harbor other health problems can experience reactive hypoglycemia after eating carbohydrates due to too much insulin release.

One of the most common reasons I see hypoglycemia occur is poor dietary choices. Foods that are high in carbohydrates and low in fat and fiber can be digested very quickly. This causes blood sugar levels to spike, and as soon as the cells use the sugar, an individual's blood sugar drops considerably. Here, an individual's blood sugar runs too low, and either the person goes back to the kitchen for another unhealthy and high-carb snack, or his or her body goes into a state of "fight or flight," releasing more cortisol triggered by the stress of low blood sugar.

Hyperglycemia

In contrast, hyperglycemia is elevated blood sugar. While hyperglycemia is much less dangerous in isolated situations, it's extremely common due to the excessive amounts of sugar consumed in typical diets today. Ongoing hyperglycemia puts a person at risk for type 2 diabetes and the many complications that accompany chronically high blood sugar.

After a meal that includes any kind of carbohydrate, your blood sugar will increase. If everything goes smoothly, your cells will absorb enough sugar, and the body will maintain a healthy blood sugar level until the next meal. That being said, not all carbohydrates or meals are created equal. For instance, drinking a soda or orange juice with a high amount of sugar but without fiber, fat or protein to slow down digestion is very different from eating a bowl of brown rice, black beans, avocado, lettuce and salsa. In fact, those two options may have the same amount of carbohydrates, but one triggers a blood sugar spike, and the other allows a slow drip of glucose to enter circulation over a few hours because the digestive process is so much more gradual when fat, protein and fiber are digested in tandem.

Excess Sugar Turns to Fat

If you consistently consume too much sugar or your body is not metabolizing glucose well, your body will use the glucose sugars to provide energy for cells and then store excess glucose as glycogen in the liver and muscle cells. Glycogen is your body's reserve fuel in case you run out of gas between meals or at night.

However, at a certain point, these storage cells will reach their maximum capacity. Imagine that you're preparing for a road trip and you stop to fill up your gas tank at the station. First, you fill up until the main tank is full. However, you have some extra cash, so you fill up the little red reserve container and put it in your trunk. You still have a few more bucks, so you decide to top off your tank. However, your tank is already full, so the gasoline starts spilling all over the ground.

This is the problem with consuming too much sugar; your system begins to spill excess energy into the bloodstream and organs. Luckily, your body has a mechanism for managing this spill. Your liver will turn sugar into fat and release that fat back into the bloodstream. The fat will be packaged with excess sugar in the blood and form a triglyceride. Triglycerides are then stored in fat cells, which is called adipose tissue. However, fat cells can also hit their max capacity, leading these little molecules to lodge into organs that they don't belong in such as the liver and muscle cells.

This is the biological process that leads to fatty liver disease and encourages excess LDL cholesterol and an increased risk of cardiovascular disease. A person who continually has dysregulated blood sugar will usually have elevated triglycerides and irregular blood glucose levels. This is a recipe for disaster and has many negative health consequences for the body.

Throughout the following pages of this book, I will continue to build on your understanding of why and how the body tries to balance blood sugar and why this might be causing your unwanted symptoms. I will also break down the relationship between imbalanced blood sugar and many of the most common chronic health conditions that are present today. If you're knowingly or unknowingly suffering from symptoms related to imbalanced blood sugar, this book will arm you with a thorough understanding of how to begin healing your body and the motivation to start now!

NOTES

CHAPTER 3

The Blood Sugar & Inflammation Spiral

JACK'S STORY

Jack is a successful man, by all accounts. He runs a large and profitable company, has a beautiful family, and until recently, had stayed active and fit. Though, at just 55 years old, he was experiencing significant neurodegeneration in his legs, progressively losing his ability to stand steadily and control his movements.

Over the years, intense stress, eating junk food on the run, and pushing through low energy with caffeine, had led Jack to a state of illness that he could no longer ignore. In addition to the worsening muscular decline in his legs, overwhelming brain fog was impairing his ability to make crucial decisions at work. Jack had a great life, but he couldn't enjoy it!

Over the months we worked together, Jack struggled to regulate his blood sugar. He was frustrated and couldn't understand how "healthy" food was causing his blood sugar to spike. It took time for him to accept new nutrition requirements and lifestyle habits. However, when he finally let go of the foods that were sabotaging his blood sugar and causing inflammation, all of his health problems began to resolve. He earned his health back and regained his coordination and vitality. In fact, just a short while later, Jack bought a farm and has been able to maintain the farm on his own as he gained back his strength and mental sharpness.

The next step in understanding how blood sugar imbalance leads to unwanted symptoms and disease is wrapping your mind around the relationship between blood sugar and inflammation. This relationship is bi-directional. That is to say that when blood sugar is out of whack, inflammation increases, but inflammation from other sources can also sabotage blood sugar balance.

That said, whenever I have a patient who has uncontrolled blood sugar, whether generally high blood sugar or endless spikes and dips, inflammation is involved. Although, it's not as simple as pointing the finger at inflammation, because the source of inflammation can be very elusive. Everything from latent viral infections to stress, poor diet, toxic load and food sensitivities can cause inflammation, not to mention imbalanced blood sugar itself.

The Bright Side of Inflammation

While inflammation is often thought of in a negative light, it isn't all bad. In reality, without the inflammatory process, our bodies would have an incomplete defense system, leaving us vulnerable to every scrape, bruise and flu. Inflammation helps your immune system respond to infections or repair injuries.

You're likely familiar with the symptoms of inflammation like heat, redness, pain and swelling. While many injuries and illnesses are obvious, others occur beneath the surface, and you may be totally unaware. Any kind of ongoing infection or injury means that low-level inflammation has the immune system under pressure and that your health is at risk.

Think back to a time when you were very sick; it's likely that a virus or bacteria had invaded your body and infected your cells. This triggered your immune system to launch an attack on the infecting bugs. By the time you felt awful, the microbes had already multiplied and lodged in many of your previously healthy cells. If your immune system was working well, it sent out the troops to kill off the infection, but they also had to kill your infected cells and clean up all the damage and debris. That said, your immune system can't just go in and wipe everything out; it must specify which cells are infected and which cells are still healthy and must be left alone. This ability to distinguish between healthy "self" cells and foreign or sick cells is called immune sensitivity.

While you sip tea and stay in bed, your body is fighting for you. You have a fever, which is meant to kill the infection with heat, along with aches, pains, swelling and flushed skin. This is all part of the attack plan. As your body destroys the infection, toxins are released from the invader, which stimulates your nerves to feel pain. Increased blood flow and lymphatic fluid move immune cells to vulnerable areas and transport damaged cells and dead pathogens out of the body. Dilated blood vessels improve blood flow and make you red and flushed, allowing for more efficient transport to affected areas. While you lay in bed exhausted, your body is doing its best to protect you.

Whether you have a broken leg or a horrible flu, you know when you've been hit, and you know when you are feeling better. However, imagine that you're harboring a low-level infection or that you have chronic work stress that leads to less obvious inflammation 24-hours a day. You may not be stuck in bed, but you won't feel great, either. Your temperature may not be 103 degrees, but you could experience headaches, agitated sleep, muscle pain and countless other seemingly unrelated symptoms.

This is low-grade inflammation, and it just so happens to be directly connected to imbalanced blood sugar and a host of other chronic diseases.[5]

What's Behind Chronic Inflammation?

Researchers have found that people with imbalanced blood sugar have overly active immune responses, and those responses cause increased inflammation.[6] However, chronic inflammation is not only intimately related to blood sugar, it's entangled with factors like chronic or traumatic stress, environmental pollution and toxins, poor diet, food sensitivities, infections and obesity. Let's look at how these different influences trigger the body into a consistent state of alarm.

The Standard American Diet

For a person living 100 years ago, much of our food products today would be completely unrecognizable. Whether it's boxed macaroni, fruit snacks or colored cereals, food has turned into a big commercial business. Throughout the agricultural and industrial revolutions, we've gained food products, but lost much of our food's nutritional value. At its base, the meals and snacks we eat should give us energy and the nutrients that we need to function optimally. However, as food processing has become the "norm," the diminished nutritional value of food alongside increasing levels of sugar, additives and calories have completely changed the way food fuels us.

Corporate agricultural production practices focus on quantity over quality. As an example, genetically modified organisms (GMO) foods have been altered in laboratory settings to resist increasing quantities of sprayed herbicides and insecticides. This benefits farmers who want to protect their crops from insects and weeds so that they can yield more harvest each season. It's easy to understand the farmers' motivation, but the unintended consequence is food that is making us sick.

For starters, farmers practice monocropping for GMO foods instead of using traditional crop rotation, a practice that adds to the soil's nutrient density. Rich soil means more nutrients for you. Unfortunately, every year the same species is grown, the land has increasingly less vitamins and minerals that specific plant needs to grow. This nutrient deficiency means that you're getting the same number of calories from food without the nutrition provided to generations past.

Moreover, GMO crops designed in labs can withstand toxic pesticides that wipe out everything around the crop including the nutrient-producing microbes in the soil. That's right; the soil microbes actually produce vitamins as their by-product, which make their way into the crops and into your body. Worse, pesticides don't remain in soil; they travel on your produce to your fork, where you ingest them. When pesticides aren't killing pests, what are they doing to you?

Killing Your Bugs

Your microbiome (that symbiotic group of microbes that colonize your gut and promote good health) is also killed off by pesticides. In reality, your microbes are pests! Most people think that by washing their food, they're protecting themselves from exposure, but that's not the case. In fact, many pesticides are now injected into seeds before they're ever planted. That means every part of your food is toxic!

Sadly, this isn't the end of the inflammatory factors associated with nutrition. If you're already eating a 100% whole food diet, your risks with produce may end there, but most people in the US are not eating a whole food diet; they're eating a highly processed diet. After pesticide-laden crops are harvested, the degradation continues. Crops go to factories where they're turned into packaged foods. During food manufacturing processes, high heat and chemical processing denatures nutrients. Then sugar, sodium, preservatives, food dyes and other additives make your food "shelf-stable" and heighten flavors to compensate for the flavors lost in processing. By this point, your food has plenty of calories but very little nutritional value. That causes nutrient deficiency, leaving your cells starving for the building blocks they need to function well.

Plants aren't the only concern we must pay attention to. Animal products can also be extremely harmful due to practices like prophylactic antibiotic use, crowded feedlots and GMO grain feeding. These industry standards mean that the meat, poultry, yogurt, milk or eggs that you eat are saturated with pesticide and antibiotics. Worse, this food has significantly less nutritional value than a pasture-raised animal and more inflammatory fats as well. You are what you eat, and the same goes for a chicken. If your poultry isn't eating a healthy diet or getting the activity it needs, its body is inflamed and unhealthy, and that is passed on to you.

So, how does this translate into inflammation? There are two primary routes. The first is that your immune system is launched into action because your body recognizes the chemicals in your food as dangerous. Part of the immune response is inflammation, so if you're eating immune-stimulating toxins every day, your body finds itself in a vicious cycle. Sadly, many toxins store themselves in your cells, which can lead to chronic inflammation.

While your body struggles to handle the toxic load coming from your diet, more stress is put on the body. That stress means the body needs even more nutrients to function. That, unfortunately, is the second major issue of today's American diet: nutrient deficiency.

On a continuous basis, each of our bodies are performing myriad biological processes like turning food into fuel, breathing and oxygen circulation, breaking down damaged tissues and recycling the cellular components, filtering molecules out of the body to maintain fluid balance and other countless operations. The regulation of these vital tasks depends on the availability of micronutrients and macronutrients, which supply construction material and tools for every cell function in the body. When the body doesn't have a healthy ratio or amount of nutrients, these processes downregulate or stop altogether. This is where disease begins.

A very common deficiency that I see regularly is a lack of vitamin D. Vitamin D acts as a hormone and a nutrient and is involved in innumerable functions throughout the body. Your body needs vitamin D for the optimal function of cardiac muscles, bone formation, hormone and immune regulation, brain cell communication and more.[7]

So, consider what happens if you're deficient in vitamin D— your body is forced to downregulate some functions so that it can prioritize others. Let's assume that your body chooses to divert vitamin D to cardiac muscles instead of bone formation, allocating vitamin D from what it deems "less critical" to essential. Over time, you would probably develop osteoporosis and other signs of vitamin D deficiency. If your diet isn't providing everything your body needs to function, you're unconsciously negotiating these deficiencies constantly. Nutrient deficiencies decrease function, and decreased function causes cells to die and inflammation to persist.

Stress

In today's stress-addicted culture, it's hard to identify what "normal" stress feels like compared to the type of stress that causes the body to break down. The state of chronic stress most people feel is far from manageable and can lead to dysregulated stress hormone production, leaky gut and poor blood sugar control. Chronic stress has even been shown to affect genes, causing them to trigger chemical production that leads to higher states of inflammation.[8]

Obesity

The standard American diet typically results in obesity, which is another important connection to understand between diet and inflammation. One of the reasons today's diets result in obesity is that they provide too many calories.

So, why is everyone overeating? For starters, processed food is addicting due to the heightened and processed flavors. Another reason, which receives less attention, is that even if the body gets enough calories but not enough micronutrients, the brain will tell your body it's still hungry in an effort to get you to consume more vitamins and minerals. This leaves people in a condition of feeling hungry but also leaves them overfed, a condition that leads to "malnourished obesity." Excess weight results in overwhelmed fat cells, which secrete inflammatory molecules that travel throughout the body damaging tissues. Obesity is a major cause of inflammation and dysfunctional blood sugar metabolism.

However, just by losing weight, one does not stabilize his or her blood sugar. In fact, my patients are much more successful at losing weight once they stabilize their blood sugar and focus on improving their overall health. By doing that, their bodies naturally and easily lose weight!

Poor Sleep

Sleep is the body's time to regulate, clear waste and heal. Getting the right amount of good quality sleep has short- and long-term health benefits. On the other hand, regular bouts of poor sleep increase one's risk of developing imbalanced blood sugar and chronic diseases by increasing inflammatory chemicals and decreasing the methylation of genes, which instigates disease pathways.[9-10] Getting sufficient sleep increases insulin sensitivity and helps to regulate blood sugar.[11]

Feeding a Healthy Gut

In each of us, there is a unique balance of microbes such as bacteria, fungi, parasites and viruses that exist in and around us. The gut is home to a diverse microbiome that is vital to our health. Alongside healthy microbes, dangerous pathogens compete for space and resources. The balance of bugs and the strains of microbes that colonize within the gut determine much about our well-being.

Lifestyle and diet have a huge impact on the survival of healthy species that are specifically threatened by a poor diet, pharmaceuticals, toxins, stress and a list of other factors. When healthy microbes are overrun by these influences, unhealthy bugs have a chance to flourish leading to...you guessed it... inflammation! With recent scientific advances, researchers have found that these gut microbes can impact blood sugar-regulating genes and change the trajectory of disease.[12]

Toxins

Unfortunately, we can no longer trust that our local water, food and air are clean and safe. Plastics that house our food and water deposit hormone-disrupting molecules into our bodies that store in fat cells and interrupt our metabolism. An even lesser-known fact is that indoor air is filled with toxins released from the off-gassing of fire retardants on furniture, carpet and clothing. Worse, circulation of forced air in our homes often traps pollutants from vehicle exhaust and factories. These consistent chemical stressors collectively damage our bodies, change our genetic expression and increase inflammation, which sets the stage for disease.13

Infections

Chronic and often unknown infections anywhere in the body lead to consistent low-level inflammation. In fact, many chronic diseases are linked to parasite, fungal, viral and bacterial infections in and outside of the gut.[14-15] Infections put pressure on the immune system and increase physical stress. As a result, blood sugar metabolism becomes imbalanced and difficult to regulate.

Cooling Inflammation

Throughout the following chapters, you will continue to see the connection between blood sugar, inflammation and the most prevalent diseases affecting the US today. Part of an effective treatment plan is digging down to the root of inflammation. It's not enough to identify that it exists. As a practitioner, it's my job to identify the sources of inflammation in each of my unique patients and help them regulate their inflammatory responses. Because of the bidirectional nature of blood sugar and inflammation, regulating both imbalances go hand in hand when healing the body as a whole.

NOTES

CHAPTER 4

Stress &
Blood Sugar
Dysregulation

LYNN'S STORY

Lynn had experienced years of chronic stress and mounting health problems. Like many, she had seen countless doctors over the years, but few had taken her symptoms seriously. By the time she was 48 years old, she was finally diagnosed with and autoimmune disorder due to elevated antinuclear antibodies. Her doctor could not specify which autoimmune disorder she had but told her they would have to wait and see how her condition developed over time. Basically, they had to let her immune system cause irreparable damage in her body before they were willing to diagnose or treat her.

Lynn suffered severe brain fog, fatigue, painful joints and other symptoms of inflammation. We quickly began identifying foods that were pushing her blood sugar out of healthy ranges while we detoxed her liver and healed her gut. Lynn responded quickly, noticing improved mood and increased energy. Her pain began to melt away and her mind felt sharp again.

Once Lynn was back to her old self, she asked me "What condition did I have?" I replied, "I don't know, and now we will never have to find out."

W e've touched on many aspects of inflammation and how they affect the body and brain. All of these factors increase the risk of chronic disease, mental health problems, learning disabilities and blood sugar control. However, the topic of stress deserves a little more attention when we look at the relationship between blood sugar, inflammation and overall health.

In today's modern world, feeling "stressed-out" is a well-accepted state of mind for most Americans. While stress can be dangerous, it's not always bad. In fact, our ability to feel stress is responsible for keeping us alive. Acutely stressful situations, like almost falling down the stairs, trigger a response that allows us to react by increasing awareness and cognition as well as reducing the pain response.[15] In this moment, our blood sugar can shoot up, providing much needed energy to our muscles and other tissues.

On the other hand, chronic or traumatic stress does not provide the same benefits. Instead it causes detrimental changes to the body and brain, initiating a process that leads to mental and physical disease and dysfunction.[15-17]

The reality is that most of us deal with acute or traumatic stress here and there, but chronic stress affects most Americans today. The American Psychological Association published staggering statistics in 2014 revealing that over 77% of Americans now experience regular physical symptoms of stress, and over 73% regularly experience psychological symptoms of stress.18 Almost half of the country reports that stress has a negative impact on their personal and professional lives. Where is all of this stress coming from?

The leading causes of stress in the US include job pressure, money, health, relationships, poor nutrition, media overload and sleep deprivation.[19] In 2017, the future of the nation and political concerns were added to the top of the list. Because the number of people experiencing high levels of stress is so prominent, our culture has settled into believing that this is a normal and acceptable way to live. Unfortunately, our bodies have not adapted to this super-charged pace of life, and the underlying physiological repercussions of stress are leading to increasingly more symptoms of chronic and debilitating disease.

Again, because stress is so common, it's easy to ignore what this word actually means. Stress is not just a state of mind; it's a state of being that shifts the entire chemical balance within the body. The stress response has evolved to keep us alive in times of danger. Imagine living long ago when humans lived as nomads, vulnerable to attack by other tribes or even wild animals. Your small tribe may have come under attack by neighboring groups, or you may have found yourself eye to eye with an animal that wanted to make you its next meal.

In a situation like this, your body's only job was to use every resource to keep you alive and get you out of the situation. In that moment, a series of chemical reactions would have initiated to stimulate a fight-flight-freeze reaction. This chemical response occurs between the hypothalamus, pituitary and adrenal glands, which we refer to as the HPA axis.

Hypothalamus-Pituitary-Adrenal Axis

The hypothalamus-pituitary-adrenal axis, or HPA, is triggered when stress or trauma occurs. Whether physical or psychological, stress stimulates the sympathetic nervous system to begin a cascade of events. Hormones secreted from the hypothalamus stimulate the pituitary gland to release a hormone called ACTH, or adrenocorticotropic hormone. ACTH then prompts the adrenal glands to synthesize and release cortisol, your stress hormone.[20]

Hormones like cortisol communicate messages throughout the body. When cortisol is produced at the end of that cascade, cortisol acts as a feedback system telling the hypothalamus and pituitary to reduce production of the hormones that were involved in the process. The production of cortisol, in essence, signals the hypothalamus and pituitary that the "stress message" was received loud and clear. The problem with this is that the hypothalamus and pituitary are not just responsible for initiating a cortisol response. They are responsible for many functions throughout the body, so if elevated, cortisol causes them to slow down for too long and too often, leading other functions throughout the body to slow down as well.

Ready to React

Once cortisol levels are elevated, you're ready to react. Whether you have narrowly escaped a car accident, you're having an argument with a loved one or your blood sugar has plummeted, your body is stressed. However, your stress response evolved to help you get out of immediate danger, so for that moment, only certain functions throughout your body are necessary to keep you alive, and others can be put on hold.

While epinephrine, another stress hormone, prompts your liver to release stored glucose into the bloodstream (elevating blood sugar temporarily), cortisol breaks triglycerides and fat stores into fuel.[21] Along with priming the body with energy sources, stress increases heart and lung function to provide more oxygen and nutrients to muscles and other tissues that are involved in protecting you. In concert, hormones are moving blood away from areas that aren't required for survival such as the reproductive and digestive organs. Increased cortisol communicates to your body that it is NOT time to relax, reproduce or eat.

A Double-Edged Sword

While this eloquent process helps ensure safety and survival, consider how damaging this process could be if your body stays in a chronic state of stress over time. While short and intense periods of stress can promote immune system function and increase anti-inflammatory signaling, when cortisol levels are elevated long-term, inflammation increases and health-promoting hormones decrease and downregulate.[22]

This is one of the primary reasons that stress is linked to disease. Our bodies can't delineate between the threat of being eaten by a wild animal and the stress of financial problems or freeway traffic. Whether we're plagued with stress from finances, family life, work, an overwhelming schedule or trauma, the biochemical "domino effect" is the same.

While it's true that we must battle our own stress response, it's important to note that the foundation of our stress response is based on our birth mother's stress response. Scientists have found that these HPA hormone imbalances are passed down from mother to child.[23] This means your grandmother's response to stress and trauma while she was pregnant with your mother shaped the way that your mother's HPA axis developed in utero. If your grandmother experienced high stress (high cortisol), your mother's already imbalanced HPA axis could have been further impacted by trauma or chronic stress prior to your birth. That HPA pattern would have been passed on to you as you grew in her womb. So, in theory, each generation may improve or worsen the next generation's capacity to manage stress. This has a direct effect on the risk of disease.

Trauma, Chronic Stress and Your Health

Decades of research have now firmly linked stress responses to health outcomes. The effect of chronic stress on a person's health is really dependent on his or her response. Consider a person who gets cut off in traffic, shrugs and goes back to listening to his or her audiobook. Compare that response to the person who gets cut off and starts yelling, making nasty gestures and stews over the experience for the next 20 minutes.

Stress response is one thing, but trauma is another. Over the last 20 to 30 years, valuable research has helped us understand the effects of trauma on health and well-being. The Centers for Disease Control (CDC) and Kaiser California partnered to perform a study between 1995 and 1997 involving over 17,000 members who completed an eight-question survey about childhood trauma and neglect. Each ACE, or adverse childhood event, such as childhood abuses and household disruptions prior to 18 years of age increased the participant's risk of developing diseases such as diabetes, obesity, cardiovascular disease, stroke, depression, asthma, disability, severe obesity, mental distress and many other chronic diseases.[23-28] These traumas include exposures to mental illness, substance abuse, imprisonment, separation or divorce, adult violence, physical abuse and sexual abuse. The study was able to conclude that with each additional trauma experienced, an individual's risk of developing serious chronic disease increases regardless of financial or social status.

Stress and Blood Sugar

Because trauma and chronic stress increase the presence of stress hormones, which increases blood sugar, a body under stress is often vulnerable to poor blood sugar control. However, that's not the end of the story. Stress hormones increase inflammation throughout the body, and that causes cell and tissue damage.[29] Cortisol is meant to be anti-inflammatory; however, in chronic stress situations, it actually increases inflammation.[30]

This dysregulation makes cells less sensitive to cortisol and insulin, two of the primary hormones that manage blood sugar levels in the body. Hormones are means to communicate information to cells, but if the cells can't hear the message, the body loses function.

As time goes on, blood sugar becomes more imbalanced, the immune system is out of whack and inflammation grows within the body. At this point, the immune system, which is meant to respond to a threat, kill it, clean up the damage and then go back into a resting state, may be switched into the "ON" position indefinitely. The inflammatory molecules meant to protect the body now begin to cause damage instead of helping us out. One specific system that gets hit hard by stress, inflammation and high blood sugar is the gut.

Diet, the Gut and Neurotransmitters

Stress shuts down digestion, and when you mix chronic stress with imbalanced blood sugar or a high-sugar diet, it sets the stage for an unhealthy microbiome, which means you're going to experience inflammation and neurotransmitter dysfunction. This may not seem obvious, but this is a major route for the connection between blood sugar imbalance and disease.

Dysbiosis in the gut, meaning overgrowth of unhealthy bacteria or not enough healthy microbes, creates a few problems. First, unhealthy bacteria produce inflammatory molecules and toxic molecules, namely lipopolysaccharides, which are linked to cell damage and inflammation. Secondly, the microbes in your gut are responsible for the production of many neurotransmitters in your body. If you don't have enough bacteria to produce vital neurotransmitters, your brain and nervous system will suffer.

Neurons (brain cells) that run from your intestines all the way to your brain can carry the signals of neurotransmitters and inflammatory signals into the brain. One of the most well-known nerves directly damaged by high blood sugar is the vagus nerve.[31] Neurotransmitters are the communication molecules in the brain, and while some stimulate the brain, others calm neurons down. Consider the consequence of too much or too little stimulation; this might look like anxiety or depression.

Many neurotransmitters are produced in the gut by healthy bacteria, so if the population of healthy bacteria is depleted and pushed out by unhealthy species, neurotransmitter production can be depleted. This is the case with many people suffering from impaired blood sugar control. Even more surprising is that these little microbes can change the way your DNA expresses itself throughout the body and brain. These microbial modifications to DNA can lead to brain changes resulting in mental illness, learning disabilities and cognitive decline.[32]

Stressing About Stress

When my patients learn about the connection between stress, blood sugar and their health, they have a tendency to become more stressed about their stress levels. It's important to consider that stress is cumulative and that your body doesn't really distinguish between emotional stress, physical stress or environmental stress. So, wherever we can make a dent in the total stress load, we get results. While I work with my patients to reduce every major aspect of their stress, simply balancing blood sugar alone reduces stress and the subsequent inflammation. It's a great starting point and can increase energy levels so that other stressful areas of life are more manageable.

CHAPTER 5

Your Brain
on Glucose

REMEMBER SARAH?

Remember Sarah, the 40-year-old mother of three? As you may recall, when I first met her, I was deeply concerned about her neurological health. Over time, the regulation of her blood sugar helped cool the inflammation in her brain, and she began a path to neurological healing. You may be interested to know that after three months, she could stand on one foot, walk in a straight line and speak in coherent sentences.

The great majority of the patients I work with who struggle with erratic blood sugar are suffering from cognitive decline in one form or another. This is because the brain is more reliant on glucose metabolism than any other part of the body, so when things go wrong in the world of blood sugar, the brain takes a big hit.

But if sugar is so bad for us, then why do we love it so much, and why does the brain rely on it to function? The simple answer is that we need carbohydrates to live, and our brains are conditioned to lead us to the easiest sources. Humans have evolved to seek out and consume glucose-containing carbohydrates because almost every cell in the human body is dependent on glucose for fuel, but none more than the brain.

Glucose is the most simple and preferred source of energy for cells, especially brain cells. Most of our cells perform an elegant process called glycolysis (glycol=glucose and lysis= dissolving), which breaks glucose apart. From there, glucose by-products are metabolized and eventually used to create ATP, the molecule that stores and transfers energy. It's this critical process that facilitates human growth, learning, moving and functioning.

While almost all cells need ATP to function, none are more demanding for glucose than brain cells. The brain accounts for just about 2% of the body's total weight but requires a whopping 20% of the available glucose.[33] Neurons (brain cells) are insatiable for glucose because they need energy 24 hours a day just to manage the basic requirements of life like regulating blood flow and breathing. The brain's dependence on glucose is also needed for higher-level functioning such as thinking, remembering and learning. Not only do brain cells depend on glucose for their own survival but also for the production of neurotransmitters, which are responsible for communicating information between neurons. If the brain runs out of energy (or even runs too low on energy, for that matter), it cannot orchestrate the intricate functions required for a healthy life.

The Insatiable Brain

Over the span of human evolution, our brains have enlarged, therefore increasing the demand for glucose. Until agricultural and industrialized food production made processed and sugar-laden foods readily available, humans had to work quite hard to find sugar. Consider the millennia prior to the agricultural revolution when human beings were hunter-gatherers. Sugar was primarily found in wild fruits and plant sources, which are naturally low in sugar. To meet the demands of the body and brain, large amounts of plant-based foods were required for survival.[34] This served the purpose of providing healthy sources of carbohydrates and high levels of vitamins, minerals and fiber. However, that does not mean that they ate a high-carbohydrate diet. In fact, most experts conclude that our hunter-gatherer ancestors received about half of their calories from animal sources, meaning their carbohydrate intake was fairly low, making up only about 20-40% of their diet depending on the region.[35]

While humans relied on low-carbohydrate diets to survive, they knew that when they found carbs, they needed to take advantage of the energy source. Imagine heading out for your daily gathering duties and coming upon a beehive. This would have been an energy oasis thousands of years ago. In that situation, your brain would have been programmed to consume as much sugar as possible, providing energy and maybe even storing some for later (in fat cells). These giant energy deposits ensured survival for times when less energy was available in the same way that killing a buffalo may have. Most of us in Westernized cultures have access to food on a regular enough basis that our bodies no longer need to "store" energy for later. However, our brains are still programmed to do so.

For this primal reason, the brain not only triggers the physical sensation of hunger but also rewards you for consuming sugar by releasing the "pleasure" neurotransmitter, dopamine. We have evolved in such a way that we now link our consumption of sugar to enjoyment, motivating us to search it out and eat more of it. With this response, it is no wonder that many of us consume too much sugar. Unlike our hunter-gatherer ancestors, we now have sugar readily available to us in every store, kitchen and restaurant, often hiding in foods that we least expect!

The Brain – Glucose Balancing Act

You have probably experienced your brain's dependence on glucose without even knowing it. Have you ever been hungry and noticed that your concentration was waning, and you began to feel a bit "foggy?" When this happens, your brain may be running low on glucose and is unable to produce enough energy to focus. Do not worry; your brain has sophisticated mechanisms that can sense when blood sugar is low, and it reacts by sending messages to the body that it needs more energy.

Throughout this process, you may begin to feel sensations of hunger and even cravings for sugary foods. The brain is wired to look for the fastest source of fuel, so oftentimes people make the mistake of grabbing a high-sugar snack like crackers, snack bars, chips, cookies and candy. While these small bites may give the brain a burst of energy, there are problems with "quick-fix" snacks, which I will cover later in the chapter.

The body has many regulatory processes critical for maintaining balance. As I just mentioned, if the brain doesn't get enough glucose, it will begin sending nerve signals for more. The brain is so dependent on glucose that it will reduce the availability of glucose to cells like muscles and organs to ensure the survival of neurons. While the brain has mechanisms to protect against many other states of deprivation, fuel deprivation will cause cell death. If the problem is simply that a person has not eaten recently enough, a meal can remedy the problem, and the brain will recover from the little slump in energy. However, there are many more concerning reasons why the brain may not be getting enough glucose or utilize it properly even when it's available.

Just as I discussed in chapter 1, insulin is required for the uptake of glucose into the brain cells. If sufficient amounts of insulin are not available or if the receptors on the brain cells do not recognize insulin (insulin resistance), then glucose may be circulating within the brain while unable to enter the brain cells where it's converted to energy. This creates a secondary problem: too much glucose remains in circulation. If glucose cannot enter brain cells, excess circulating glucose damages cells and tissues while the brain cells starve. This is a double whammy and is unfortunately very common in cases of chronic hyperglycemia and diabetes.

Consistently high and low blood sugar are problematic for the brain for another critical reason. These two states are both known to damage the blood brain barrier (BBB).[36] The BBB is essential for keeping the brain safe. It's a selectively permeable membrane, which means that it chooses what comes in and what goes out. In essence, it's the brain's protective firewall. When this membrane is damaged, invaders can enter, and critical substances can exit. This not only affects the brain glucose metabolism and homeostasis of the brain fluid but also leaves the brain more vulnerable to infection.

Having a healthy level of available glucose for brain cells is the first step, but the brain must also be able to efficiently break down glucose into smaller subunits before it can be used for energy production. Researchers have found that people who cannot efficiently break down glucose (glycolysis) into the smaller molecules required for energy production are also at risk for brain damage and cell death. In fact, this malfunction of glucose metabolism directly links high blood sugar to Alzheimer's disease.

The Marriage of Mental Illness and Blood Sugar Balance

Physical illnesses like cancer, autoimmunity, cardiovascular disease and Alzheimer's only account for one side of the health complications that accompany blood sugar imbalance. Mental health, poor mood and learning disabilities are the flip side of glucose dysregulation. However, this connection is slightly more complex because high blood sugar is not necessarily the cause; instead, it seems that diabetes, mental illnesses and learning disabilities may be branches of the same tree.

In 2016, 20% of US kids were struggling with learning disabilities such as ADHD and dyslexia.[37] Each year, approximately 1 in 5 adults in the US experiences mental illness, and 1 in 4 diabetics suffers from depression.[38-40] Between 1990 and 2000, antidepressant prescriptions for SSRIs (selective serotonin reuptake inhibitors) increased by a shocking 1300%, and over 30 million Americans spend more than $12 billion on antidepressants annually. This is hard to fathom given that much of the research has concluded that antidepressants are no more effective than sugar pills (placebos).[41] In fact, while most healthcare providers are still blaming mental health on chemical imbalance, research is pointing to inflammation and nutrient deficiency as underlying causes of many psychological disorders.

Millions of Americans are suffering from mental health issues in tandem with other inflammatory conditions like diabetes, which makes it hard to ignore the relationship. Based on the information you learned in the last chapter connecting Alzheimer's to diabetes-induced inflammation, you know that the brain is not safe from the damaging effects of high blood sugar. Cognition, mood swings, depression, anxiety, bipolar disorder and learning disabilities all hold relationships with dysregulated blood sugar and inflammation.[42-44] In fact, our brains are vulnerable to blood sugar irregularities before we're even born. Children born to mothers with gestational diabetes are at a much higher risk of developing learning disabilities, obesity and inflammatory diseases throughout childhood and later in life.[44]

Many of the same pathways that lead to chronic physical diseases pave the way to mental illness as well, and it's not uncommon for physical and mental illnesses to manifest from imbalances that seem unrelated. For instance, hormone imbalances can result in symptoms of anxiety, depression or insomnia. Severe thyroid dysfunction can mirror bipolar disorder or invoke uncontrollable anxiety. Overgrowth of certain bacteria within the digestive tract can reduce the production of neurotransmitters, leading to depression or anxiety symptoms.

Moreover, research suggests that insulin resistance could be caused, in part, by elevated levels of hormones linked to depression.[45] Even common vitamin and mineral deficiencies can provoke symptoms of mental illness. In fact, a vitamin B3 deficiency is a well-known cause of severe anxiety, while a magnesium deficiency is a known cause of insomnia.46 These are just a few examples of how the web-like connections throughout the body link unlikely but related conditions. So, what's going on beneath the surface that marries blood sugar imbalance and mental health problems? You guessed it— it is largely due to inflammation.

When inflammation is prolonged, there's a higher risk of depression, anxiety and blood sugar fluctuations. However, insulin resistance, anxiety and depression are also thought to increase inflammatory chemicals in the body, perpetuating and exacerbating symptoms and disease progression. This means that high blood sugar does not necessarily cause depression and other mental health issues; instead, it seems they can both set the stage for the other. In fact, adolescent depressive symptoms are linked to poor insulin control in adulthood.[12] It is a vicious cycle of inflammation, imbalance and disease.

NOTES

CHAPTER 6

The Diabesity
Epidemic

SAM'S STORY

Sam was 62 when we met and had been struggling with high blood sugar for over a decade. Years of stress, confusion about how to eat well and mounting prescriptions had left him exhausted, frustrated and at his wits' end with healthcare providers.

Sam was currently taking 3 prescriptions for blood sugar, one of which was injectible. Even with all of the drug therapy, his HbA1c was still stuck at a dangerous 6.3.

Sam explained that he tried to eat a "healthy" diet, but his doctors had been telling him for years to eat whatever he wanted and to control his unstable blood sugar with drugs.

Contrary to his conventional doctors' approach, we began to monitor how his body reacted to his typical meals. We quickly found foods that his body could not handle, and within only 6 weeks, his fasting glucose levels upon waking were down to 72, a sign that he needed to stop taking drugs that were lowering his blood sugar.

Just a couple of months later, Sam was able to maintain blood sugar levels between 80-100 with diet alone. His HbA1c dropped under 5.7, and he had lost 10 pounds. Sam was no longer diabetic and no longer a slave to prescriptions.

W e can't discuss blood sugar without diving into diabetes, the epidemic that's sweeping the globe. Over the past few decades, billions of dollars have been allocated to understanding sugar metabolism, and for good reason. Type 2 diabetes has hit epidemic levels with more than 30 million Americans (almost 10%) harboring this dangerous disease, and 1/4 of those are living with it unknowingly.[47] It's estimated that over 54% of the population will have diabetes by 2030.[48] To add to this concern, over 84 million Americans are on their way to an initial diagnosis of prediabetes, which untreated, will develop into type 2 diabetes.[47] The National Diabetes Statistics report found that under 12% of people living with prediabetes knew that they had it.[47] By 2030, it is estimated that annual medical and social costs will rise to over $622 billion.

These figures are pretty shocking given that diabetes is completely preventable and even reversible in many cases, and so are the conditions that most often exist alongside it. In fact, diabetes rarely exists as a stand-alone diagnosis; it is most often compounded with obesity and metabolic syndrome, leading many doctors to refer to this condition as "diabesity."

Even with staggering numbers like these, conventional healthcare is doing little to prevent or successfully treat diabetes. In fact, it is expected that 1/3 of adults will have diabetes by 2050, many of them developing it in childhood.[49] Currently, almost 200,000 kids have type 2 diabetes.[50] More shocking is that 18.5% of kids in the US are obese, putting them at significantly higher risk of developing type 2 diabetes throughout their lifetimes.[51]

What are the Symptoms?

While diabetes can exist without overt obesity, it almost always accompanies abdominal obesity, often referred to as a muffin top or spare tire. This relationship is not only physically obvious but also reveals itself in lab results such as:

- **dyslipidemia (low HDL, high LDL and high triglycerides)**

- **high blood sugar (fasting above 100 mg/dL, Hb1Ac above 5.5)**

- **systemic inflammation**

- **high blood pressure**

Even without lab results, many people know something is "off" due to symptoms such as:

- **sugar cravings, especially after meals**
- **·sugar cravings that aren't relieved by eating sweets**
- **fatigue after meals**
- **frequent urination**
- **increased thirst and appetite**
- **difficulty losing weight**
- **slowed stomach emptying**
- **sexual dysfunction**
- **visual problems**
- **numbness and tingling in the extremities**

Although some symptoms may seem unrelated to diet, each of these irregularities is a sign that your body is unable to effectively use food for fuel and that damage is occurring beneath the surface.

Branches of the Diabetes Tree

Both type 1 and type 2 diabetes are familiar to most people, and it's likely that we all know someone who is struggling with one of these conditions. Type 1 diabetes is an autoimmune disorder that occurs when a person's immune system attacks and damages the pancreatic beta cells that produce insulin. Type 2 diabetes is a non-autoimmune condition caused by insulin resistance and high blood sugar, rendering the body inefficient at using carbs for fuel!

However, in addition to the typical manifestations of diabetes, there are three lesser-known forms of diabetes that receive very little attention or treatment. Many people that don't fully identify with either category are most likely suffering from poor blood sugar control without proper diagnosis or treatment!

Prediabetes

Prediabetes can be likened to the calm before the storm... something isn't right, but you aren't exactly sure what it is.[52] Often, when patients realize their blood sugar is a little high (100 and 125 mg/dl), they are grouped into the prediabetic range. Many doctors will put them on Metformin or tell them to eat "healthier" and cut out sugar! Conventional practitioners rarely, if ever, search for the root of what's causing the imbalanced blood sugar.

No one becomes diabetic overnight. When a blood sugar imbalance isn't corrected at the source, the body becomes more inflamed and insulin resistant, which can lead to metabolic syndrome. After years of imbalanced blood sugar, it's not surprising when a patient develops full-blown type 2 diabetes.

Type 1.5 Diabetes

A less familiar variation of diabetes is type 1.5 diabetes. Type 1.5 means a person has a combination of types 1 and 2, so autoimmune factors and insulin resistance are driving the blood sugar imbalance.53 Patients who are diagnosed as adults are often assumed to have type 2 diabetes and aren't properly tested for a concurrent autoimmune disorder. Some of these patients may inject insulin every day, but each time they do, their immune systems attack the insulin as an invader. This is one reason some patients are unable to manage their condition much less improve it.

Type 3 Diabetes

Increasingly more evidence links imbalanced blood sugar to Alzheimer's disease each day. In fact, this relationship is often referred to as type 3 diabetes![54] People with diabetes have twice the likelihood of developing Alzheimer's. In fact, obesity and metabolic syndrome alone can lead to cognitive dysfunction. Alzheimer's is no longer believed to be a complication of diabetes; instead, the two appear to develop from a shared pathway that disrupts the immune system and leads to inflammation throughout the body.

Dr. Dale Bredesen, an internationally recognized expert on cognitive health, aging and Alzheimer's has spent decades uncovering the disease pathways that lead to brain disease and decline. He has classified "types" of Alzheimer's based on these pathways.[55] One pathway involves chronic inflammation, which may be rooted in a number of imbalances that cause an imbalanced immune system and high levels of circulating inflammatory molecules. A second pathway involves non-inflammatory imbalances such as insulin resistance or vitamin deficiencies.

However, Dr. Bredesen has identified the "combo deal," which is when a person exhibits both pathways, which is often the case with diabetics. This should make sense based on what you now know about blood sugar imbalance and inflammation. Inherently, any blood sugar imbalance will not only affect the fuel source for brain cells but also increase the presence of inflammatory molecules that damage neurons. This means that you DO NOT HAVE TO HAVE DIABETES to be at risk. Your brain is at risk if your blood sugar regularly spikes and dips.

The Obesity, Diabetes and Metabolic Syndrome Triad

While carbohydrates and blood sugar take the spotlight when it comes to diagnosing and treating diabetes, blood sugar is not the major problem for diabetics. In fact, high blood sugar is merely a symptom. While this symptom is independently dangerous to one's overall health, fixing an individual's blood sugar does not fix the disease. This is apparent because even when pharmaceuticals successfully lower blood sugar levels, diabetics do not get better. In fact, they progressively decline and experience devastating complications such as neuropathy, loss of limbs, blindness and increased risk of other terrifying diseases. If I want to know why my patient has developed diabetes, I must dig deeper than blood sugar or poor diet.

The truth is that not everyone who is overweight has diabetes, and not everyone with diabetes is overweight. This is not a simple disease, and there are always other factors involved. Often, there are trends and one of them is the relationship between obesity, metabolic syndrome and dysregulated blood sugar.

There is no singular path to developing this triad. In truth, all of these can occur as standalone illnesses that are unrelated to the others. However, I usually find that when one of these illnesses develops, the others are not far behind.

My patient, Andrea, is a great example of how these disorders develop in tandem and as a sequence. Andrea grew up in a small agricultural town in Iowa. While her family was not involved in farming, her neighbors were growing crops such as wheat and corn. She ate a very standard American diet steeped in processed and high-sugar foods. When she was young, she was very thin and active, but her eating habits were cemented over those years, so by the time she went to college, she was about 20 pounds overweight.

Let's pause for just a moment and look at how Andrea's upbringing may have influenced her diabetes development. Research is clear that toxins, including those used in agricultural practices, increase inflammation and disrupt proper hormone signaling.[16] Those influences alongside a diet that lacked micronutrients but was flushed with antibiotics, additives, pesticides, unhealthy fats and sugar created a foundation for imbalance, deficiency and toxicity. Although Andrea was not technically "obese" upon entering college, she was holding a lot of extra weight around her belly. These fat cells produce chemicals that increase inflammation and interfere with hormone signaling. At this point, Andrea was unknowingly on the road to disease.

Throughout college, she suffered the normal stresses of school and continued to put on weight. However, between her junior and senior year of college, she lost her best friend in an auto accident and experienced deep trauma and depression throughout her last year of school. By now, she was 35 pounds overweight and beginning to suffer the early signs of diabetes and hormone imbalance. She struggled to sleep, she could not lose weight no matter how much she restricted her calories and her menstrual cycle was very irregular. She felt fatigued and craved sugar all day.

After she graduated, she had a health exam for her new job, and the labs indicated that she was prediabetic with high triglycerides and LDL. Her doctor put her on metformin to control her blood sugar and suggested she eat a low-fat diet. At this point, her cells were already struggling to use carbohydrates for fuel, and while the metformin lowered her blood sugar levels, it did little to increase her insulin sensitivity and her disease continued to progress. She was feeling worse by the day, exhausted and unfocused. She was developing chronic pain and could not keep up with her other 23-year-old friends. On weekends, she was sleeping over 12 hours every night and never felt rested.

Unbeknownst to Andrea, inside her body, excess fat cells were stimulating the production of more and more inflammatory molecules. Her cells were becoming more resistant to insulin, and glucose was struggling to enter her cells for fuel production. While she was restricting her fat intake, her body was manufacturing excess fat from the never-ending supply of glucose that was circulating in her blood. Fat cells were getting filled to their max, and fat was beginning to deposit in her liver and muscles cells, impairing function and leading to more inflammatory molecules and chronic pain. Her body was starving for fuel while she was gaining weight.

By the time I saw Andrea, she was 35. She came to me with every symptom of metabolic syndrome and had already developed full-blown diabetes. She was taking daily insulin injections and was tired of feeling awful every day. Her doctors were only able to offer her drugs and ineffective dietary advice. In Andrea's opinion, she had tried every diet, fitness plan and miracle drug, but nothing helped her lose weight or improve her energy.

In Andrea's case, we began monitoring her blood sugar and identifying what foods and meals were derailing her. Within two weeks, we identified the carbs that she could not tolerate and increased her fat and fiber intake to keep her blood sugar stable between meals. Within three months, Andrea's A1c had dropped to 5.4, which is below the prediabetic range. She had lost 20 pounds and was raving about her energy levels. This is not a miracle; this is what I see every time my patients work to establish good blood sugar control!

Andrea has a relatively "classic" diabetes story. Not everyone follows this trajectory. In fact, I have had patients who started off with high blood pressure and high cholesterol and became overweight and diabetic over time. I have also had patients who were diabetic and not visually overweight. The term for this condition is "metabolically obese," and often, these patients are storing excess fat in and around their organs. I have had patients that were prediabetic for 20 years without shifting into full-blown diabetes but suffered many of the metabolic abnormalities that a diabetic person experiences.

The point is that there is no one picture of diabetes, diabesity or metabolic syndrome. To that end, some obese people will never develop diabetes, although they may suffer from other metabolic complications. The problem of diabesity is almost too big to wrap our heads around, and it currently affects more than one billion people worldwide.[47]

Dangers of Diabetes

Diabetes may make you fatigued and overweight, but that is not what makes this such a serious disease. The real problem is the internal damage diabetes perpetuates. Imbalance and inflammation are at the root of diabetes. This means that your body is getting too much of (or not enough of) something. For example, this can mean that you have too many toxins and not enough antioxidants and nutrients to naturally detox. This can mean too much sugar and not enough micronutrients. This could mean too much food in general or trauma and chronic stress. Identifying the source(s) of the problem is critical to stopping the disease, but it is only the beginning. As time goes on, imbalances in the body affect other systems which then start to unravel and affect other systems, and the web of dysfunction continues.

For instance, you may not know that your body requires cholesterol to repair damaged cells or build new cells. Cholesterol is part of the cell membrane. Let's assume that there is an underlying source of inflammation damaging cell membranes throughout the body. This damage is going to affect insulin receptors and other receptors on the cells' surface. Now we have the beginning of insulin resistance because the cell can't receive insulin efficiently. Glucose will begin to collect in the blood, and the liver will do its best to package it into triglycerides to lower blood sugar levels. We also have the compounding issue that the cell is being damaged and will require more cholesterol to fix it, so this will trigger the liver to generate more cholesterol. At this point, we have an insulin-resistant person with high triglycerides, high blood glucose and high cholesterol.

This is just one example, but my point is that insulin resistance and diabetes set the stage for other risks that include cardiovascular disease, neuropathy, blindness, limb loss, cancer and more. Once chronic damage is triggered in the body, it cannot be resolved with blood sugar management alone. The entire picture needs to be accounted for and dealt with. Blood sugar is a problem, but I see it as the "canary in the coal mine" and not the end of the story. Well before full-blown diabetes evolves, escalating blood glucose levels are telling us that something is going on.

Conventional medicine is still treating diabetes as the only blood sugar problem of our era. Worse, conventional practitioners are treating blood sugar problems as the cause instead of the symptom of something much deeper. In reality, most of my patients struggle to regulate blood sugar, but very few have diabetes. In fact, their lab results almost always look normal. That's because we are testing the average blood sugar level (HbA1c) over three months. However, the test does not necessarily tell us how well they are managing blood sugar throughout the day or in response to different foods.

By focusing on diabetes as the only "problem" associated with blood sugar, we're missing the subtle warning signs that come well before that diagnosis. We also risk missing the people that are suffering from dysregulated blood sugar whose conditions will never develop into diabetes but will result in other devastating diseases. It's true, your blood sugar does not lie, but we have to be willing to listen.

CHAPTER 7

The Vicious **Cycle**

PATTY'S STORY

Patty had been fighting high cholesterol for years. She had recently celebrated her 60th birthday and was becoming increasingly concerned about her stubborn cholesterol levels, which were hovering around 250 in total. Concerned with the side effects of statins, she had continually declined her doctor's recommendations to start prescription therapy. Instead, she opted for natural supplements and a bowl of oatmeal each morning, a remedy she had read was helpful for lowering LDL cholesterol.

I explained to Patty that imbalanced blood sugar often increases cholesterol. In fact, the liver produces more cholesterol in an attempt to repair damage often caused by high blood sugar-related tissue damage.

Once Patty began monitoring her blood sugar, she was shocked to find out that her cholesterol-lowering breakfast routine was, in fact, sabotaging her blood sugar. Her glucose levels were spiking to over 150 after each bowl.

After Patty learned the foods that were spiking her blood sugar, she was able to stay in a healthy blood sugar range and her cholesterol dropped to 200. She went off all cholesterol supplements and no longer lives in fear of the risk factors associated with high cholesterol.

D iabetes is far from the only condition related to imbalanced blood sugar and inflammation. Arthritis, autoimmunity, high cholesterol and cancer are among the list of diagnoses that are directly related to uncontrolled glucose levels, but that's not all. It turns out that dysregulated blood sugar and insulin imbalances are intricately connected to all chronic diseases. In many cases, out-of-whack blood sugar steers the body towards illness, but sometimes existing illnesses bring about insulin resistance and blood sugar problems. Much like the relationship between inflammation and blood sugar, many chronic conditions make it hard to pinpoint where the disease began. One thing we do know is that regulating blood sugar is imperative to correcting each of the illnesses we are about to dive into.

Just like the swelling diabetes epidemic, diseases like autoimmunity, hormone dysfunctions, Alzheimer's, cardiovascular disease and cancer are increasing at alarming rates. Unlike injuries or infections with a "known" cause, these diseases are chronic, and their origins are complicated, complex and often unknown. This poses an especially difficult problem for conventional medical doctors who treat symptoms instead of the underlying source of disease because their training does not usually prepare them to identify the root but only to manage the disease. As a result, trillions of dollars are spent on chronic disease "management" each year, but patients never recover; instead, they steadily get worse.

Unfortunately, the foundation that conventional medicine was built on does not support the prevention or effective treatment of chronic disease. In my grandparents' time, it was normal for doctors to make house calls, but even throughout my childhood, I could rely on my doctor to remember what grade I was in and which sports I played. Now, the norm for doctors is to rush patients through the office and quickly treat a diagnosis based on a list of symptoms. This in-and-out style of care happens for a few reasons: doctors are not trained to identify the root cause of chronic disease, and they are pressured by insurance companies to see way too many patients each day to cover their overhead.

Sadly, we are in a new era of illness that conventional medicine has not adapted to. While the US is the leader in medical spending throughout the world, we ranked a pathetic 43rd in life expectancy in 2014. In fact, healthcare spending for chronic diseases account for 90 cents of every dollar spent on healthcare in the US. In 2011, this amounted to $2.3 trillion of the $2.7 trillion spent.[56] These statistics mean that we are not effectively addressing the largest causes of disease and death in our country.[57]

We're just not doing enough to prevent and reverse the most predominant causes of death in the US: heart disease, tobacco-related and colon cancers, COPD, Alzheimer's disease and other forms of cognitive decline. Despite spiking medical costs, these largely preventable and lifestyle-based diseases are stumping policy makers and healthcare giants. It is hard not to question whether there is an intentional disregard for the science that can direct us to effective treatment and prevention.

A staggering number of Americans— over 59% of the population— are directly affected by one or more chronic diseases; a cost to our nation of over $42 trillion between 2016 and 2030. On every front, these diseases are winning. In fact, between 1990 and 2016, deaths from lifestyle-based hormone, metabolic, blood and immune disorders increased by almost 90%.[58]

It is not as though conventional medicine doesn't see the problem clearly; conventional practitioners just don't know how to fix it. The World Health Organization (WHO) admits that 80% of premature cases of heart disease, stroke and type 2 diabetes, and over 40% of cancers are completely avoidable if Americans stay away from tobacco, follow healthier eating habits, and are more physically active.[56] The CDC agrees, stating that "The United States cannot effectively address escalating health care costs without addressing the problem of chronic diseases." In other words, we are obviously doing something wrong.

Let's be clear, though. The real issue with chronic disease is not death— we are all going to die. The problem we are facing, and the costs associated, are the decades of illness and poor quality of life that come before people pass away. There are countless years wasted between wellness and death for most Americans. Most of my patients can't remember what "good health" feels like or the last time they felt it. Most report that childhood or young adulthood marked the end of being comfortable in their bodies.

I usually tell my patients who are struggling with one or more chronic diseases that my responsibility as their doctor is to help them live a long and healthy life and then "drop dead." Of course, this is an outrageous statement, but behind this comment's shock value is a question; would you like to glide into your golden years in a nimble body that allows you to move and think freely, or would you like to endure exhausting symptoms of disease for decades until you are finally too worn out to carry on? The conversation is meant to illustrate a point: aging does not have to mean illness, and we have a choice. We all want to feel fit until our 100th birthday and then fade away painlessly in our sleep. My job is to help my patients achieve a full life of health and skip the years of suffering.

Unfortunately, this fate is the exception and not the rule. One reason it's not the typical reality is that the medical community has an unexplainable resistance to treating the complexities of chronic disease with attention to the interconnectedness of your systems. We can't simply state that a patient has imbalanced blood sugar and throw medication at him without digging deeper into how blood sugar is affecting the immune system, hormones, metabolism and the like. It's crazy to separate the systems as though they somehow each exist in a vacuum.

Much like the coupled and bi-directional relationship between blood sugar and inflammation, chronic diseases that are responsible for our healthcare crisis are deeply intertwined with how we eat, move and live. Blood sugar affects and is affected by the most prevalent chronic diseases. We must use blood sugar not only as a diagnostic tool but also as a warning sign and starting point for all other chronic disease. Let's look at the major diseases affecting people today and see how blood sugar is involved.

Autoimmune Disease

Dr. Datis Kharrazian is a leading expert in autoimmune conditions such as Hashimoto's thyroiditis, the primary cause of low-thyroid conditions. In his groundbreaking book Why Do I Still Have Thyroid Symptoms When My Lab Tests Are Normal, he discusses some of the critical relationships between blood sugar and autoimmunity. Probably the most important takeaway is that every time your blood sugar spikes or dips, tissue damage occurs. This means that if your body is regularly in a state of blood sugar imbalance, injury is constantly plaguing your healthy tissue, leading you into chronic inflammation and often autoimmunity.

Autoimmune disease is an umbrella term for disorders that develop when the immune system attacks healthy tissues throughout the body. The immune system mistakenly identifies healthy cells as invaders and does what it is designed to do— to launch an inflammatory response for destruction and repair. Of course, when you're actually injured or infected with a virus or bacteria, this is a very helpful process; however, if your immune system targets healthy tissues, this becomes a big problem.

Autoimmune conditions are far-reaching and still not fully understood. The immune system can turn on any tissue, leading to very different symptoms even though the root immune dysfunction is the same. Conditions such as rheumatoid and psoriatic arthritis, Hashimoto's thyroiditis, multiple sclerosis, type 1 diabetes and ALS are all based in autoimmunity. The symptoms should not be the focus, though. We should shine the spotlight on the symphony of root causes. This is where blood sugar takes center stage.

Autoimmune diseases are multifactorial, meaning the disease has no singular cause but many possible influences. In fact, there are countless options for the imbalances and conditions that contribute to autoimmunity, but Dr. Alessio Fasano, a leading expert in autoimmunity has found three commonalities among those suffering from autoimmunity: genetics, environmental triggers and intestinal permeability. So, how do these three factors relate to blood sugar?

Genetics

The fact is that your genes can put you at an increased risk of having imbalanced blood sugar, autoimmunity and any other chronic disease, but in order for your genes to turn on you, they need to be triggered. Overt factors like smoking, stress, poor diet or heavy metals can turn on the genes that trigger inflammation and blood sugar problems, but imbalanced blood sugar can also stimulate a genetic shift towards promoting autoimmunity. Therefore, having uncontrolled blood sugar puts people at a higher risk of developing an autoimmune condition. The stress and inflammation caused by unregulated blood sugar means that the immune system is not only navigating obvious injuries and infections but also trying to constantly repair the damage caused by high blood sugar. When this is ongoing, your worn-out immune system can't keep up, and healthy tissues are at risk.

Intestinal Permeability

The intestinal permeability component muddies the waters even more. Around 70-80% of the immune system originates in the gut.[59] This makes a lot of sense because cells within the intestines are gatekeepers to your delicate system on the other side of that intestinal wall. The digestive tract not only has to identify potential dangers to digestion and absorption but also must break down the healthy elements, like nutrients, and transport them across the intestinal barrier into the bloodstream. This is a complicated and heavy job!

Intestinal permeability is a problem in individuals with autoimmunity and dysregulated blood sugar. A diet high in sugar and refined carbohydrates can feed unhealthy microbes, cause the intestines to break down and result in undigested food and pathogens gaining access to circulation. That triggers the immune system even further and leads to food sensitivities, as the immune system recognizes the undigested food particles as invaders. Of course, that leads to higher inflammation and worsening blood sugar control.

Consuming a high-sugar diet and having imbalanced blood sugar can increase the risk of developing an autoimmune disorder, but it does not just flow one way. Having an autoimmune condition means increased inflammation, and we already know that inflammation means damage to insulin receptors, which leads to insulin resistance and poor blood sugar control. To successfully treat imbalanced blood sugar or autoimmunity, we must consider both systems and how they interact.

Environmental Triggers

Environmental triggers include psychological stressors, trauma, toxic exposure, infections, dietary trends and more. These factors can stimulate genetic vulnerabilities and propel the body into a state of disease. Understanding the different environmental triggers that each person has experienced throughout his or her life can be crucial for identifying the best therapies to calm the inflammatory response and set the stage for healing.

Hormone Imbalances

Hormones are chemical messengers that direct functions throughout the body. Often, we think of hormones as estrogen, testosterone and progesterone, but those are only sex hormones. Endocrine glands throughout your body produce a variety of hormones that regulate stress, hunger, metabolism, mood, libido and more.

It's important to know that hormones are carried throughout the bloodstream until they find their target cell. They know they have arrived when they fit into the receptor on the cell's surface, just like a lock and key. When a hormone fits into a receptor, it triggers a specific function. This means that the glands, hormones and receptors must all be working well for your hormones to balance. Many factors can throw hormones out of whack such as stress, toxins, poor diet, obesity, diseases and the like. There are so many relationships between blood sugar and hormone function that this topic is the subject of countless books and thousands of research articles.

I want to give you an example so that you can begin to understand this relationship. Consider my friend Marita. She went through a very stressful period in her thirties, which resulted in years of poor sleep, bad dietary choices and too much caffeine and alcohol. Throughout the five years that she was dealing with difficult personal problems, she put on about 30 pounds. She constantly felt achy and tired and soon found out that she had developed insulin resistance and, therefore, high blood sugar. If we pause at this point, we can begin to create a hypothesis around why this may have happened.

Marita may have had a genetic risk for blood sugar imbalance or any other inflammatory condition. She may have even had underlying infections or toxins that were affecting her immune system. One thing we know for sure is that under chronic stress, her adrenal glands were pressured to produce the stress hormone cortisol. Cortisol helps us manage acute stress and keeps us in the "on" position, but over time, cortisol increases inflammation, reduces insulin sensitivity and interferes with thyroid function. It's also directly involved in blood sugar regulation, called on to increase blood sugar when it gets too low. So, Marita's stress led to risk factors related to inflammation, thyroid disorder and blood sugar dysregulation. She was not supporting herself with good nutrition, quality sleep, stress management skills or exercise, so her body was growing increasingly more dysfunctional by the day.

When she first visited her primary care doctor, he discovered that her blood sugar fell into prediabetic range and told her to lose weight. The problem was that he did not test her thyroid thoroughly, and her attempts to lose weight were made nearly impossible by a failing thyroid. We know that insulin resistance increases the risk of thyroid disorders, but doctors often fail to make this connection.[60] To make matters worse, receptors on her cells had been damaged by the inflammation so her cells were not efficiently receiving insulin, thyroid hormone and cortisol leaving her body to run on empty. As I said, Marita is a friend, so I was not comfortable treating her, but she was so fed up with the vicious cycle she was in that she eventually saw one of my colleagues who discovered that Marita had also developed low estrogen. So, she had a range of hormone imbalances that were resulting in a chronic inflammatory process and a host of miserable symptoms. While this all seems overwhelming, the bottom line is that her blood sugar was affecting (and being affected by) the hormones throughout her system. Without addressing every imbalance, she was not going to get her life back.

Androgen Imbalance

Sex hormones like estrogen and testosterone are also at risk of being thrown out of balance when your blood sugar is off. A blood sugar imbalance leads to stress, which means too much cortisol is required for daily functioning. When the body requires a lot of cortisol, sex hormones take the hit. This is why.

Pregnenolone is the precursor hormone to both cortisol (by way of progesterone) as well as estrogen and testosterone (by way of DHEA). If day after day your body is trying to make enough cortisol to keep you going, it is stealing resources from sex hormone production.

Moreover, cortisol increases aromatase activity, which in men, causes testosterone to convert to estrogen. Men who are experiencing a high conversion rate of testosterone to estrogen will experience symptoms like:

- **Increased fat mass**

- **Lower libido**

- **Low mood and energy**

- **Insomnia**

- **Increased cardiovascular risk**

- **Prostate problems**

Men with this imbalance will often exhibit female characteristics such as breast tissue and fat around the hips.

In women, stress (caused by imbalanced blood sugar or other sources) does not cause a testosterone–estrogen conversion but instead causes the overstimulated adrenal glands to produce too much testosterone. This is often seen in women suffering from polycystic ovary syndrome and in that case is usually linked to insulin resistance. This can result in symptoms like:

Hair loss on the scalp

Excess body hair (especially upper lip, chin, chest and abdomen)

- **Infertility**

- **Acne**

- **Oily skin**

- Increased body odor

- Sleep disturbance

- Irritability, aggression and other mood changes

On the other hand, increased cortisol has also been linked to estrogen dominance, which can yield symptoms like:

- **Hair loss**

- **Thyroid dysfunction**

- **Sluggish metabolism and weight gain**

- **Foggy thinking, memory loss**

- **Fatigue**

- **Trouble sleeping/insomnia**

- **PMS**

- **Low libido**

- **Irregular or otherwise abnormal menstrual periods**

- **Bloating (water retention)**

- **Breast swelling and tenderness**

- **Fibrocystic breasts**

- **Headaches (especially PMS-related)**

- **Mood swings (most often irritability and depression)**

- **Cold hands and feet (a symptom of thyroid dysfunction)**

It is important to keep in mind that hormones and blood sugar are intertwined on every level. We cannot treat blood sugar without treating hormones, and vice versa. Remember that insulin is a hormone and when it is out of balance, other hormones follow suit. It is also critical to understand that we cannot just look to hormones for answers; we must know that the glands that produce them and the cells that receive them are healthy too.

Debbie was convinced that she was fated for a future of fatigue and brain fog after overcoming thyroid cancer but losing her thyroid gland in the process. Her hemoglobin A1c was high, indicating that she was suffering from type 2 diabetes. At 54 years old, she lacked energy, motivation, passion and vitality, making every day feel like an uphill battle. She was already dealing with a tricky thyroid balancing act, but with her blood sugar out of whack, I knew there was no way her energy would ever stabilize.

Almost as soon as we started monitoring Debbie's blood sugar, she became empowered and excited. Before long, she was bringing in intricate graphs and spreadsheets that tracked her responses to the dietary changes she was making. Debbie "owned" this process and took personal accountability for every step.

Cancer

High blood sugar increases the risk of several cancers and reduces the effectiveness of treatment. In fact, diabetes increases the risk of developing liver, pancreatic, bladder, breast, colorectal, esophageal, biliary tract and endometrial cancer as well as lymphoma by up to 200%.[61] Cancer is an area of constant and extensive research, so we do not have the full scope of how this devastating disease operates in every situation.

What we do know is that a diet high in sugar, obesity and having high blood sugar increases the level of advanced glycation end products (AGEs) throughout the body. AGEs of advanced glycation end-products are little molecules that develop when proteins are exposed to sugar. AGEs increase damage and inflammation throughout the body and cause premature aging and chronic disease.[62] AGEs are also thought to play a role in the increased damage caused to vascular tissue in diabetics.

To make matters worse, high insulin—a characteristic of high blood sugar— is known to be carcinogenic and act as a growth factor for cancer.[61] We know that cancer cells are insatiable for glucose; they use it for fuel to help them grow and proliferate. When cancer is in a high-sugar environment, it can grow bigger even when elevated insulin is not a factor. This means that a high-sugar diet or any form of high blood sugar can feed the strength of cancer.[63-65]

Cardiovascular Disease

According to the American Heart Association, 68% percent of people over 65 years old with diabetes die from heart disease, and 16% die from a stroke. I hate to sound like a broken record, but we must look at why this is happening, and the arrows point to inflammation yet again. We have established that inflammation comes before insulin resistance and imbalanced blood sugar. Remember that inflammation is a normal immune process that is caused by what your body recognizes as an illness or injury. Cardiovascular diseases (CVDs) are also inflammatory in nature, so we can think of high blood sugar and CVDs as two branches of the same tree. Having either of these conditions pours gasoline on the fire of inflammation within the body, helping it to spread. Many people don't know that cholesterol is produced in the liver to repair damage throughout the body, so elevated cholesterol can be a sign of ongoing damage.

Dysregulated blood sugar means that your body is inflamed, but it also causes damage to the vascular system, leaving blood vessels in need of repair (cue the cholesterol) and inflammatory processes on high alert. All of this means that more insulin receptors on cells are damaged, sugar can't enter cells and blood sugar keeps getting higher. When glucose damages areas in the blood vessels, immune cells and cholesterol collect in that area causing blockages, often referred to as plaque. This means a heart attack or stroke is likely to follow. Plaque and inflammation cause your blood vessels to lose flexibility, which results in high blood pressure and a higher risk of CVDs; the cycle spirals out of control. We need to look at high blood sugar as a symptom of inflammation and a warning sign for CVDs.

Alzheimer's Disease

Accumulating research has concluded that the same insulin resistance behind blood sugar dysfunction may also be a significant mechanism in the development of the memory-disrupting plaque seen on the brains of people with Alzheimer's.[66] Some studies have even found evidence of this plaque in the pancreas of patients with type 2 diabetes, linking these two diseases.[67]

Researchers have linked inflammation caused by chronically elevated blood sugar to damage in brain tissue. I am running the risk of sounding like a broken record, but this goes back to inflammation again. High blood sugar damages brain cells and the small capillaries that bring oxygen and nutrients to the brain, all the while brain cells die from starvation because glucose can't get in to fuel them. This whole dysfunctional situation alerts the immune system to send help. An inflammatory process is launched to clean up the dead brain cells and damaged tissue. In many people, the inflammatory structures that are characteristic of Alzheimer's called amyloid plaques are not broken down after they do their job. They remain in the brain and interfere with neuron communication and blood flow, leaving more brain cells to die and brain function to be lost. You don't have to have diabetes to have inflammation from imbalanced blood sugar. If your blood sugar levels are fluctuating all day, your brain is at risk.

Insulin resistance and poor blood sugar control are not the only routes to Alzheimer's, but they are two major routes and areas of deep interest. High blood sugar and its counterpart high insulin are intertwined with all chronic disease risks. What is less clear is the totality of the impact that this can have on the relationship between the two.

Many of these diseases can negatively impact blood sugar, and blood sugar can set the stage for any of these common chronic diseases to develop. As doctors and patients, we need to make sure that we are looking at all factors to give the body the best chance at preventing and healing disease. As you now know, these diseases do not develop in isolation they manifest in concert with each other.

CHAPTER 8

Blame it on
Your Genes

BREE'S STORY

Bree had been diabetic for years, and while she took metformin daily, her HbA1c still hovered around 7.7. At 53 years old, Bree knew her risk of developing other diseases was growing as long as her blood sugar remained high. Bree had a family history of poor blood sugar metabolism, and we had already worked with her mom, helping her reverse diabetes.

Over the following three months, we helped Bree identify foods that caused her blood sugar to spike and dip while designing a menu that stabilized her blood sugar. In just 90 days, her HbA1c sunk to 5.7, dropping her out of the diabetes range. As a bonus, Bree lost 20 pounds without increasing activity or changing any other aspects of her life. She beamed as she reported that her energy was high, her brain fog gone and her motivation to continue healing was strong.

When I am working with patients, they are seldom concerned with statistics, labels or symptoms; the question they want answered is "Why?" Why did their bodies fail them by losing the ability to metabolize carbohydrates? Unfortunately, there is no one-size-fits-all answer that will apply to everyone. As I explained in the previous chapters, the common theme among people who do not efficiently metabolize carbohydrates is inflammation.

Inflammation can be caused by many factors such as chronic stress, trauma, poor diet, infection, obesity and exposure to toxins through pollution or heavy metals. Most of my patients have suffered a combination of these influences, and when mixed with certain genetic variations, the body loses optimal functioning and disease develops. Regardless of what has caused the dysfunction, when a person cannot utilize carbs but continues to consume too many or the wrong ones for his or her body, inflammation increases, and it perpetuates a vicious cycle.

Is it Bad Genes?

Most commonly, my patients have a preconceived notion that their genes are driving their illnesses or symptoms. Genes are always a factor, but they're far from the whole story. A common saying in functional medicine is "Your genes are the gun, but it's your environment that pulls the trigger." In essence, your genetic code can make you vulnerable to disease, but environmental exposures and lifestyle choices will help determine whether these genes will turn on and trigger disease progression. For example, although offspring have a high probability of inheriting type 2 diabetes (25-80%), genes account for only 10% of this risk; the majority of the risk lies in the habits passed down by parents.[68]

Within the last few decades, the growing field of epigenetics has revealed that lifestyle choices and environmental exposures can activate or silence helpful and hurtful genes. When genes are "turned on," they express proteins involved in cellular structure, hormone communication or any number of important molecules that keep you alive and functioning. On the other hand, genes that are switched off stay silent. "On" genes serve as the instruction manual that tells your body what to make and how to function.

Now, consider a friend or acquaintance who smokes, has a poor diet, drinks too much liquor and sits around on the couch all day. These habits can turn on genes that code for disease. But if that old friend makes a dramatic lifestyle shift, switching to an organic diet, daily yoga classes, an occasional glass of red wine and annual meditation retreats, his or her genetic code (DNA) would be exactly the same, but the genes that are turned on and sending the instructions would change completely. Epigeneticists confirm that healthy lifestyle habits like these can turn on the genes that prevent disease and turn off the genes that are working against you. More importantly, your lifestyle changes can influence how your genes direct your health!

NOTES

CHAPTER 9

THE **SECRET** SAUCE

REVERSING EMBALANCED BLOOD SUGAR

B y now you know that living with blood sugar imbalances means that your body is in danger and in need of deep healing. You also know that managing blood sugar is about more than guesswork, carb-counting, broad-spectrum health advice and prescriptions. Instead, you must give your body every available resource to halt the inflammatory process and reverse the damage that has been done. This chapter is a general but thorough guide to balancing blood sugar.

That being said, I strongly advise that you work under the care of a functional medicine provider to help you navigate the "bumps in the road," tailor your therapies to meet your individual needs and provide laboratory tests to monitor your progress. In my clinic, not only do I work with each of my patients to balance his or her blood sugar but also work alongside a skilled nutritionist who helps each patient navigate his or her individual dietary needs. It is that important for healing! However, you don't need to wait for your first appointment to begin balancing blood sugar. You can start NOW!

Track Your Blood Sugar Patterns

Just about every one of my patients uses a blood sugar monitor for a period of time to identify their blood sugar patterns. It's critical to log trends in blood sugar throughout the day to give you and your provider feedback on how to better support your body with the tools below. Measure your blood sugar when you wake, before each meal and 45-60 minutes after each meal. We ask our patients to check their blood sugar 3-4 hours after each meal, as well, but that often aligns with their pre-meal check.

It is equally important to keep a diary of your blood sugar levels, what you ate, how you slept, your energy levels throughout the day and your bowel movements. All of this information helps your provider make connections between your symptoms and your blood sugar.

As I've shared, most of my patients have specific foods that cause their blood sugar to dip or spike. They may also have some carbohydrate-rich foods that they can metabolize well but others that throw their blood sugar out of whack. The trick is finding those patterns by tracking meals and blood sugar until you've established the meals and foods that keep you balanced.

Maximize the Healing Power of Nutrition

The saying "you are what you eat" could not be truer. Each step in this guide is important, but nutrition is the essential foundation of reversing a blood sugar imbalance and cannot be understated. Every bite you take should be dense with nutrients that support your body. Wasting calories by eating foods that don't deliver the nutritional bang for your buck is like throwing money down the drain.

Moreover, nutrition is extremely individualized. Those with uncontrolled blood sugar often unknowingly suffer from food allergies and sensitivities. Those foods may cause your blood sugar to respond by spiking or dipping.

I strongly advise that you work with your functional medicine provider to identify food sensitivities while making improvements to your diet. This is crucial because you may have sensitivities to healthy foods that you eat regularly, but by keeping them in your diet, you'll continue to stimulate your immune system and prevent healing. Once you identify the foods that are working against you, the following guidelines will be more effective.

Energy Availability

Your body and brain need consistent energy availability to keep you feeling sharp and balanced. Mood swings are linked to hyper and hypoglycemia because dramatic shifts in energy availability stress the body by leaving it in an energy surplus or energy deficit too often.[69] If you think back, you can probably remember a time when you were extremely hungry and began to feel the sensation that many now refer to as "hangry." This is because your blood sugar had dipped a bit too low and your body was feeling uncomfortable sensations like stomach pain, brain fog and low energy. You probably also experienced irritability and other symptoms of crankiness.

While this happens to all of us from time to time, chronically high blood sugar means that your body is fighting too hard to balance high and low blood sugar throughout the day. As you know from previous chapters, the hormones insulin and cortisol are involved in this process. Both hormones will drive up overall inflammation when they are chronically high. We've talked a lot about inflammation already, but it is a big player in setting the stage for imbalanced blood sugar and mental health problems.

General Nutrition Guidelines

Avoid Processed Food

Nutrition is extremely individual-based, but you should start by removing processed foods. Processed foods are low in nutrients and increase inflammation. Soda, cookies, candy, cakes and alcohol are more obvious culprits, but even bread (of all kinds), pasta, rice, potatoes and corn cause blood sugar to soar and provide little benefit. Even starchy vegetables like peas, squash and yams can bother some people and can contribute to unhealthy alterations to glucose levels.

While processed foods are convenient, they're also at the root of chronic disease, void of nutrients and high in sugar and calories. Processed foods are laden with additives and toxins such as pesticides. Insecticide residue on processed and nonorganic foods attack healthy microbes in the gut. Ultra-processed foods, which are so common in the current American diet, are implicated in increasing the risk of chronic disease and forcing the body into a pro-inflammatory state. To make matters worse, processed foods are extremely low in nutrient content, yielding a malnourished state even when plenty of calories (energy) are consumed.

While choosing whole foods may mean a little more time in the kitchen, it also means a little more time on this earth! Eating quality foods like organic produce and wild or pasture-raised meats means that you are giving your body what it needs and protecting it against harmful toxins. It is not easy or cheap, but it's one of the best places that you can allocate your time and money!

More on Carbs

Let me reiterate, the amount of carbohydrates in a specific food may have less to do with your blood sugar regulation than you think. However, understanding the basics of carbs can help when you're testing foods out. In general, there's a big difference between consuming 25 grams of carbohydrates from an apple and consuming 25 grams of carbohydrates from a bag of chips or candy. An apple and junk food both contain carbohydrates that can be broken down into sugar and fuel for your brain, but an apple has the bonus of containing water and fiber.

Fiber and water, along with fat and protein, serve to slow down digestion. This means that as the digestive system gradually breaks down fiber, water and sugars, little bits of sugar enter the bloodstream over time, providing a steady source of fuel. All the while, the fiber and water that remains in the digestive tract breaks down slowly and tells your brain that you're still full. As a bonus, your apple is full of vitamins and minerals that keep you healthy and vibrant.

In comparison, imagine that you chose a snack of potato chips or gummy bears to get you through your 3pm slump. This food has very little fiber, water, healthy fat or protein to slow down digestion. While you may consume exactly the same amount of sugar as you did by eating the apple, the sugar will reach your circulation quickly, causing your blood sugar to spike. The body must scramble to deal with the excessive amount of fuel, secreting insulin and trying to shuttle it into cells throughout the body. However, if the glucose metabolism is impaired in any way, which is often the case for those who eat processed foods regularly, then sugar may linger in the bloodstream instead of fueling the intended brain cells. In addition to this problem, the processed food snack is laden with unhealthy additives and void of vitamins and minerals that the body needs to stabilize blood sugar and support other vital functions.

It's also important to consider the quantity of food you're eating to earn those carbs. To consume about 25 grams of carbs in an apple, you get to eat about 200 grams of food, or one large apple. To consume the same amount of sugar in gummy bears or chips, you only get to eat about 50 grams of food. Let's break it down: 50 grams of potato chips is ½ of a single-serving bag, while 50 grams of gummy bears is about 18 pieces. Which one do you think keeps you satiated longer? That junk food snack is not going to fill you up for long, and after your blood sugar spikes and subsequently drops, you'll likely be searching for another snack or meal before long!

Choosing healthy sources of carbohydrates that also provide you with nutrients and fiber is the first step to uncovering your route to blood sugar balance. However, if you're already suffering from impaired glucose metabolism, even a healthy carb may not be able to efficiently provide energy to your brain cells. You may need to refocus on a more primal way of eating.

Be a "Hunter-Gatherer"

Typically, a "hunter-gatherer" or Paleo diet plan is best for those with imbalanced blood sugar. This diet focuses on proteins and healthy fats, specifically wild, organically-raised or free-range animal proteins like chicken, beef, turkey, lamb, eggs and fish. Healthy plant-based fats like avocados, olives and raw nuts and seeds are also emphasized, along with plenty of non-starchy vegetables. At least 80% of the mass of your diet should be plant-based to ensure that you're consuming enough fiber and micronutrients. This means loading up on vegetables, low-sugar fruits, nuts, seeds and plant-based oils. This diet excludes grains, legumes and dairy.

The Keto-Alkaline Diet

Some patients have benefited greatly from taking their nutrition beyond general recommendations, shifting their bodies away from a reliance on glucose and into a state of using fat for fuel. This is called ketosis, and under supervision from a healthcare professional, it can do wonders for reversing high blood sugar and diabetes.

You may have heard of the ketogenic diet because it has become popularized over recent years for everything from managing chronic disease to weight loss, but the ketogenic diet is not new. In fact, it has been used for almost a century in the successful treatment of epilepsy, with no apparent side effects. Over the last few decades, the ketogenic diet has improved many conditions including autism, bipolar disorder, Parkinson's disease, multiple sclerosis, diabetes and more.

Some of its success is thought to be a result of the ketogenic diet's ability to increase the production of a very important molecule called NAD+.[70] This molecule supports energy production within the mitochondria of cells and is deficient in those with chronically high blood sugar.[71] This exacerbates the primary energy problem for those with imbalanced blood sugar - a reduced ability to use carbs for fuel. Ketones provide an alternative fuel source that increases and improves mitochondrial metabolism.[72]

When done correctly, the keto diet also provides increased intake of polyunsaturated fats. Diets high in polyunsaturated fats are linked to a reduced risk of developing all chronic diseases.[73] When eating a keto diet, most of the caloric intake is from fat, often as high as 80-90%. Foods like avocado, healthy oils, butter, meat, eggs, seafood, cheese, fatty nuts (like pecan and Brazil) and non-starchy vegetables are promoted, while fruit, grains, beans, lentils and starchy vegetables are excluded.

I think it's important to mention that my clinical experience has emphasized the effectiveness of a ketogenic diet for patients with imbalanced blood sugar. Though, as I said initially, every person is unique, and therefore, therapeutic dietary approaches for imbalanced blood sugar vary from person to person. I have seen many patients find success by eating a very low-carb diet where about 80% of their calories came from fat, while others were more successful incorporating more protein and getting between 60% and 70% of their calories from fat.

Another important distinction is that my patients who are most successful and experience better health tend to eat diets that are mostly plant-based. While there is definitely a place for wild and grass-fed meats and eggs, sources of fat such as avocado, coconut, nuts, seeds and healthy oils should form the foundation of a healthy keto diet.

Intermittent Fasting

For some, intermittent fasting can help reduce inflammation and increase insulin sensitivity.[74] It's the most popular form of fasting because it takes advantage of the sleeping hours and then tacks on an additional six to eight hours without food. In this case, people usually fast for 16 hours (skipping breakfast) and eat for eight hours throughout the day. While no food is allowed during the fasting period, clear liquids like water, tea and coffee are allowed. Intermittent fasting is linked to weight loss and reduced disease occurrence. Intermittent fasting reduces inflammation and increases insulin sensitivity; both effects lead to benefits for those struggling with blood sugar imbalance.

As a bonus, intermittent fasting has the advantage of increasing brain-derived neurotrophic factor or BDNF.[75] BDNF promotes neurogenesis, or new neuron growth.[76] BDNF also prevents cells from going through a normal biological process called apoptosis (programmed cell death) instead of keeping neurons alive.[77] If that's not impressive enough, BDNF also promotes and maintains learning and memory by protecting the synaptic areas between neurons while also safeguarding neurons from injury and infection.[78] This is specifically important for those with high blood sugar because elevated glucose levels damage and destroy neurons throughout the body. Low levels of BDNF are associated with risk for peripheral neuropathy and lower cognition, a common side effect of high blood sugar.[79] For that reason, higher levels are beneficial, while lower levels throughout the body and brain are linked to degenerative brain diseases.[80-81] For all of these reasons, I utilize the most effective techniques for increasing my patients' levels of BDNF when aiming to repair the brain.

Probiotics

Probiotics are healthy bacteria that can be taken in supplemental forms. Probiotics enter the digestive tract as a backup infantry that is tasked with supporting the healthy microbes that are competing for resources in your gut. Probiotics can help push out toxic microbes and restore your intestinal integrity and gut function. Researchers are continually working on identifying strains that effectively treat a myriad of conditions, and science is pointing to unique properties within each strain. Some bacteria that are identified as being most beneficial in restoring gut function and supporting immunity are various strains of Bifidobacterium and Lactobacillus.[82-84] Your functional medicine doctor can tailor your probiotic treatment to your specific condition.

Prebiotics and Fiber

Reinoculating a healthy microbiome is supported by feeding and nourishing healthy microbiota. Prebiotics are fibers that have been identified as capable of feeding healthy bacteria while not benefiting toxic microbes. This makes prebiotics especially valuable in balancing the biome.

Foods like bananas, onions, chicory root, garlic, asparagus, jicama, leeks, Jerusalem artichoke, yacón and blue Agave are all good sources of prebiotics. Increasing your intake of prebiotic foods is helpful, and supplementation can also improve outcomes. Supplementing with prebiotics should be done gradually and with caution if you are experiencing symptoms of small intestinal bacterial overgrowth (SIBO), as prebiotics can exacerbate symptoms.

Increasing any type of fiber can be very effective for regulating blood sugar. Because fiber slows digestion, it helps regulate the speed at which sugar can enter the blood. This alone can help prevent spikes and dips throughout the day.

Eat Regularly

Eating a healthy breakfast with a balance of protein, healthy fat and complex carbohydrates from whole foods can be extremely beneficial for your attention span and a balanced mood. Research shows that when children struggling with attention disorders experience a drop-in blood sugar (hypoglycemia) below <75 mg/dL, they experience a significant decrease in cognitive behavior and performance. Hypoglycemia can occur when a person hasn't eaten for a long period of time, such as after a night of sleep, but it can also occur from a biological response called reactive hypoglycemia. This occurs when a person eats a high-sugar/refined carbohydrate meal, forcing a strong insulin response after the blood sugar shoots up quickly and then drops too low. For this reason, it is imperative that anyone trying to maintain a balanced blood glucose level or address mental health issues eats plenty of healthy anti-inflammatory fats, plant fibers and lean protein regularly throughout the day.

Lifestyle Guidelines

Brush Your Pearly Whites

While we focus a lot of attention on the microbes within the gut, the mouth is also home to a variety of microbiota that work to keep your tissues and teeth healthy. In fact, those with gum disease have an increased risk of experiencing insulin resistance, inflammation and blood sugar dysregulation.[85] There is a "domino effect" of unhealthy pathogens in your mouth compromising the microbiome within the gut. Using charcoal and probiotic-based toothpaste is a healthy alternative to commercial brands.

Sleep

After diet, sleep is one of the most important habits for maintaining good health. Sleep offers the right condition for your body and mind to repair and restore themselves.[86] When you don't get enough sleep, your body does not have ample opportunity to perform its renewal processes, which are crucial to your overall health. Insufficient sleep decreases insulin sensitivity after only two nights of poor sleep and is linked to a higher risk of developing diabetes.[87-88]

Quality sleep is another way to increase BDNF. Over time, chronic sleep deprivation decreases levels of BDNF, likely due to ongoing elevated levels of cortisol, a common side effect of sleep deprivation.[89] Interestingly, melatonin supplementation can prevent the depletion of BDNF in sleep-deprived people.[90]

Exercise

Most people can benefit from increasing their activity level, even if it's something as low-impact as taking a long walk each day.[91] In fact, many of my patients don't have the cellular energy for an intense fitness routine, which would do more harm than good. I usually advise my patients to start slowly and increase their activity levels as they have the energy to do so. If you are currently living a sedentary lifestyle, you may choose to consult your functional medicine provider before getting started.

There are many benefits of exercise. For starters, it can reduce inflammation, regulate blood sugar and reduce the risk of developing virtually every chronic disease.[92] Exercise also reduces stress and has even been shown to regulate gene expression.[93] Exercise is helpful for promoting healthy gene expression while tamping down the expression of disease-promoting genes.

HIIT and Healing

A significant amount of research has emerged over the last decade about the benefits of a specific style of exercise called high-intensity interval training (HIIT). HIIT is a form of cardiovascular interval training that alternates between short periods of intense anaerobic exercise, aiming to reach 75-90% of an individual's max heart rate with low-impact recovery periods. Although this pushes your body to a max heart rate, because it is done in short bursts, many patients find it much less strenuous than 30-60 minutes of cardiovascular activity. There's no exact HIIT workout design or session duration, but people typically alternate between 30-60 seconds of max intensity and 30-60 seconds of recovery for 10-20 minutes depending on fitness level. This can be done with a jump rope, squats, push-ups, sit-ups, lunges, etc.

There are many benefits of HIIT such as building muscle and losing fat in a short period of time, increasing your metabolism, improving your heart health and boosting your mood. It is also a great way to use up blood sugar, lowering overall levels.

One of the most interesting benefits of HIIT workouts is that it increases a protein called BDNF, which can build new neurons throughout the body. This can be very important for those who have suffered imbalanced blood sugar because neurons are often destroyed as a result.

When consistent high-intensity aerobic exercise is compared to HIIT, higher increases in BDNF are achieved with HIIT.[94] After a single exercise session, BDNF drops back down to normal levels within ten minutes of completing the workout; however, after only six weeks of HIIT, stable BDNF levels are increased.[95]

Stress Management

As you know, chronic stress causes a series of hormonal changes that negatively affect the immune system, increase inflammation and reduce the ability to metabolize glucose. Learning how to utilize tools like meditation, deep breathing, yoga and Qigong will condition your mind and body to deal with stressors with less physical damage.[96] Yoga and meditation practices are also linked to increased BDNF, and this improvement occurs alongside better cortisol regulation and increased immune function.97

Hydration

Hydration helps your body efficiently deliver nutrients to your cells and excrete toxins and waste! Most fluids do not contribute to hydration. Coffee, tea, soda, juices and other beverages do not count towards your daily hydration since the additives in those beverages change how your body processes the liquid and have the potential to dehydrate you! Instead, increase your intake of purified water, drinking at least half of your body weight in ounces each day (150lb. person=75 oz. H2O).

Detoxification and Liver Support

The prevalence of environmental pollutants, heavy metals, pesticides and household chemicals (xenobiotics) that are deemed "endocrine disruptors" is a well-supported factor behind the explosion of diabetes and other chronic diseases within in our population. Skilled functional medicine providers use advanced testing and therapy to identify toxins, remove them and repair the tissues they have damaged. I have found that many of my patients who have "hit a wall" in their recovery benefit significantly from detoxification therapies and liver support. However, this should not be done without medical supervision.

Bodywork

If you have imbalanced blood sugar and are dealing with weight control issues, it's even more imperative to maintain the health of your muscles, joints and connective tissues. Excess weight puts added stress on your joints, and inactivity can cause your muscles to deteriorate over time, making it harder to be active and healthy. Investing in bodywork such as massages, physical therapy, chiropractic therapy and acupuncture during this period may help you recover physically.

Support System

I can't overstate the importance of having a support system by your side to help guide you through the ups and downs of your healing process. Regardless of your health status, try to surround yourself with healthcare providers, friends and family who advocate for you and support you. We typically ask that our patients bring their partners or family members to their appointments so that the people within their support systems gain an understanding of how important lifestyle changes are to the recovery process. If your family and social circle are struggling with similar health issues, I strongly suggest finding a support group or a social group that inspires you such as a hiking or swimming group.

Supplementation

While eating a whole food and nutrient-dense diet is crucial, people with blood sugar imbalances may have additional nutritional needs due to the stress their bodies are under. High-potency supplementation provides essential micronutrients and plant extracts that act as therapies for the body to help it balance and heal, typically without the unwanted side effects of pharmaceuticals. Again, I strongly advise supervision from a skilled provider. Utilizing therapeutic doses tailored to your needs is how you will get the most benefit.

Another word to the wise - it's important to buy reputable therapeutic-grade brands. Time and again, consumer watch groups have discovered that chain stores such as GNC, Walgreens and Target. often aren't selling quality supplements. Often, the supplements aren't even what they're represented to be. Use brands that your doctor recommends and that have been tested for quality.

These four supplements are well-supported by scientific research to benefit people suffering from dysregulated blood sugar.

Vitamin D

While vitamin D is a considered a vitamin, it's also a hormone that is critical for signaling and supporting countless functions within the body. Vitamin D has been referred to as the conductor of the orchestra of functions within the body. It's required for everything from calcium absorption to immune function. Low levels are linked to increased inflammation, osteoporosis, depression, cognitive decline, autoimmunity, cancer and more.[98-102] Not surprisingly, vitamin D deficiencies have also been linked to poor glucose control, and when diabetics supplement vitamin D, their glucose metabolism tends to improve.[103] Those with imbalanced blood sugar may need more vitamin D than a healthy individual due to the stress and inflammation throughout their body.

Vitamin D should be taken in conjunction with vitamin K2 (which helps to move calcium from the blood into bones). Combination supplements that contain both vitamins are available. The dosage varies based on the level of deficiency, but most adults can safely take up to 25000 IU per week. Vitamin D can be synthesized within the skin with sun exposure; however, most people do not spend enough time in direct sunlight to produce a sufficient amount. Vitamin D can also be consumed in cod liver oil, fatty fish and fortified foods. However, therapeutic doses are necessary when supporting diabetes, so supplementation is often a better option than sun or food. Vitamin D levels should be monitored, and healthy levels range from 50-80 nmol/L.[104]

Melatonin

Melatonin is a naturally occurring hormone produced by the pineal gland. Melatonin is responsible for regulating sleep cycles, so levels should be highest at night. Typically, people with type 2 diabetes have lower levels of circulating melatonin, which may lead to insomnia.[105] While supplemental melatonin is popular to improve sleep, it has additional benefits for those with imbalanced blood glucose. Poor glucose control leads to the increased production of free radicals that damage cells and promote disease. Studies have found that melatonin acts as an anti-inflammatory agent, regulating the production of specific free radicals called reactive oxygen species (ROS) in diabetes.[106] The same studies also found that melatonin protects pancreatic beta-cells, which are responsible for producing insulin and are often damaged as blood sugar dysregulation progresses. Most people find that they can tolerate 3-5 mg per night before bed.

Alpha-Lipoic Acid

Poor blood sugar control increases the risk of cardiovascular disease, neurological disorders and neuropathy, in large part due to high levels of inflammation and oxidative stress. High blood sugar impairs blood flow by reducing the production of nitric oxide in vascular tissue, therefore reducing the flexibility of the cardiovascular system. Alpha-lipoic acid (ALA) is a powerful antioxidant, referred to as the universal antioxidant, with insulin-like and anti-inflammatory activity. Studies have shown that supplementing with ALA improves insulin sensitivity and can help reduce the risk of cardiovascular disease and neuropathy in diabetics.[107-108] ALA can be found in spinach, broccoli, tomatoes, green peas, Brussels sprouts, rice bran and the organ meat of a cow. However, for therapeutic doses, it is best to use a high-quality supplement. Adults can usually tolerate ALA in doses ranging from 600-1000 mg/day.

Magnesium

Magnesium is a mineral that is so critical to the function of the human body that it has been widely studied and found to be involved in over 300 reactions throughout the body. One of those vital processes is the metabolism of ATP, the molecule responsible for energy storage within cells. In fact, magnesium is the fourth most plentiful mineral in the body, but unfortunately, most people are deficient due to poor diets and reduced magnesium content in crop-growing soil.[109]

Magnesium is required for the control of muscular contractions, blood pressure, cardiac function, vascular tone, nerve transmission and neuromuscular communication. Magnesium is also required for the proper metabolism of insulin and glucose, so it is not surprising that people with imbalanced blood sugar tend to be magnesium deficient.[110]

Low levels of magnesium have been associated with several chronic diseases such as Alzheimer's disease, insulin resistance and type 2 diabetes mellitus, hypertension, cardiovascular disease, migraines and attention deficit hyperactivity disorder.[111] Good dietary sources of magnesium include cooked greens like spinach and Swiss chard, dark chocolate, almonds, pumpkin seeds, avocado, figs and banana. However, most people can safely take 300-600 mg/ day, and many prefer to take it at night, as it helps to relax muscles.

THE TIME IS NOW

Now you're armed with the information to take control of your blood sugar and your health. The first step is monitoring your glucose levels and finding the right provider to help you make sense of them. From there, you can dig into the other imbalances that aren't fostering your best health. This is a different type of healthcare approach; it requires personal responsibility and taking ownership over your health. However, I can tell you that the rewards are great. Reversing symptoms, preventing disease and gaining years of wellness are worth the effort. I hope this book has helped to inspire you and open your mind to the possibility of living your best life. My sincerest wishes for your successful healing.

Dr. Ben Galyardt
Owner of F8 Well Centers &
Pioneer of the Galyardt Method

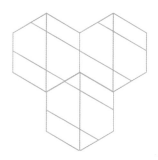

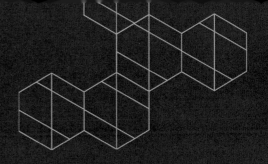

BLOOD SUGAR
DOESN'T LIE

How Hidden Blood Sugar Imbalance Drives

Chronic Disease and Brain Disorders –

and Your Guide to Fixing It!

f8wellcenters.com

References

1. Slavin JL. Dietary fiber: Classification, chemical analyses, and food sources. *J Am Diet Assoc.* 1987;87:1164-1171.

2. Slavin, J.Fiber and Prebiotics: Mechanisms and Health Benefits. *Nutrients.* 2013; 5(4): 1417-1435; doi:10.3390/nu5041417

3. Smith, P. M., Howitt, M. R., Panikov, N., Michaud, M., Gallini, C. A., Bohlooly-Y, M., ... Garrett, W. S. The microbial metabolites, short chain fatty acids, regulate colonic Treg cell homeostasis. *Science.* 2013; 341(6145).

4. Gerard Clarke, Roman M. Stilling, Paul J. Kennedy, Catherine Stanton, John F. Cryan, Timothy G. Dinan; Minireview: Gut Microbiota: The Neglected Endocrine Organ, *Molecular Endocrinology.* 2014; 28(8): 1221–1238.

5. Stranges S, Rafalson LB, Dmochowski J, Rejman K, Tracy RP, Trevisan M, and Donahue R P. Additional Contribution of Emerging Risk Factors to the Prediction of the Risk of Type 2 Diabetes: Evidence From the Western New York Study. *Obesity.* 2008;16:1370-1376. doi:10.1038/oby.2008.59

6. https://www.scientificamerican.com/article/inflammatory-clues/

7. Giovannucci, E. Expanding Roles of Vitamin D. *The Journal of Clinical Endocrinology & Metabolism.* 2009; 94 (2):418–420

8. Alcocer-Gomez E, de Miguel M, Casas-Barquero N, Nunez Vasco J, Sanchez-Alcazar JA, Fernandez-Rodriguez A, and Cordero MD. NLRP3 inflammasome is activated in mononuclear blood cells from patients with major depressive disorder. *Brain Behav Immun.* 2014; 36: 111-117.

9. Irwin MR, Olmstead R, Carroll JE. Sleep Disturbance, Sleep Duration, and Inflammation: A Systematic Review and Meta-Analysis of Cohort Studies and Experimental Sleep Deprivation. *Biological psychiatry.* 2016;80(1):40-52. doi:10.1016/j.biopsych.2015.05.014.

10. Massart R, Freyburger M, Suderman M, et al. The genome-wide landscape of DNA methylation and hydroxymethylation in response to sleep deprivation impacts on synaptic plasticity genes. *Translational Psychiatry.* 2014;4(1):e347-. doi:10.1038/tp.2013.120.

11. Leproult R, Deliens G, Gilson M. Beneficial impact of sleep extension on fasting insulin sensitivity in adults with habitual sleep restriction. *Sleep.* 2015 May 1; 38(5):707-15.

12. Brunkwall L, Orho-Melander M. The gut microbiome as a target for prevention and treatment of hyperglycaemia in type 2 diabetes: from current human evidence to future possibilities. *Diabetologia.* 2017;60(6):943-951.

13. Collotta M, Bertazzi PA, Bollati V. Epigenetics and pesticides. *Toxicology.* 2013;3 (307): 35-41

14. De Luca C, Olefsky JM. Inflammation and Insulin Resistance. *FEBS letters.* 2008;582(1):97-105. doi:10.1016/j.febslet.2007.11.057.

15. Charmandari E, Tsigos C, Chrousos G. Endocrinology of the stress response. *Annual Review of Physiology.* 2005; 67:259–284.

16. Smith SM, Vale WW. The role of the hypothalamic-pituitary-adrenal axis in neuroendocrine responses to stress. *Dialogues in Clinical Neuroscience.* 2006; 8:383–395.

17. Levine AB, Levine LM, Levine TB. Posttraumatic stress disorder and cardiometabolic disease. *Cardiology.* 2014; 127:1–19. DOI: 10.1159/000354910

18. https://www.stress.org/stress-research/

19. Stephens MAC, Wand G. Stress and the HPA Axis: Role of Glucocorticoids in Alcohol Dependence. *Alcohol Research : Current Reviews.* 2012;34(4):468-483.

20. Padgett, David; Glaser, R (August 2003). How stress influences the immune response. *Trends in Immunology.* 24 (8): 444–448. doi:10.1016/S1471-4906(03)00173-X. PMID 12909458.

21. Thomas JC1 Letourneau N, Campbell TS, Giesbrecht GF; Apron Study Team. Social buffering of the maternal and infant HPA axes: Mediation and moderation in the intergenerational transmission of adverse childhood

experiences. *Dev Psychopathol*. 2018 Aug;30(3):921-939. Doi: 10.1017/S0954579418000512.

22. Padgett, David; Glaser, R (August 2003). How stress influences the immune response. *Trends in Immunology*. 24 (8): 444–448. doi:10.1016/S1471- 4906(03)00173-X. PMID 12909458.

23. Chanlongbutra A, Singh GK, Mueller CD. Adverse Childhood Experiences, Health Related Quality of Life, and Chronic Disease Risks in Rural Areas of the United States. *Journal of Environmental and Public Health*. 2018;2018:7151297. doi:10.1155/2018/7151297.

24. Talbot J., Szlosek D., Ziller E. Research & Policy Brief. Portland, Me, USA: University of Southern Maine, Muskie School of Public Health, Maine Rural Health Research Center; 2016. Adverse childhood experiences in rural and urban contexts.

25. Gilbert L. K., Breiding M. J., Merrick M. T., et al. Childhood adversity and adult chronic disease: An update from ten states and the District of Columbia, 2010. *American Journal of Preventive Medicine*. 2015;48(3):345–349. doi:10.1016/j.amepre.2014.09.006.

26. Brown D. W., Anda R. F., Tiemeier H., et al. Adverse Childhood Experiences and the Risk of Premature Mortality. *American Journal of Preventive Medicine*. 2009;37(5):389–396. doi: 10.1016/j.amepre.2009.06.021.

27. Felitti V. J., Anda R. F., Nordenberg D., et al. Relationship of childhood abuse and household dysfunction to many of the leading causes of death in adults: the adverse childhood experiences (ACE) study. *American Journal of Preventive Medicine*. 1998;14(4):245–258. doi: 10.1016/s0749-3797(98)00017-8.

28. Hostinar CE, Lachman ME, Mroczek DK, Seeman TE, Miller GE. Additive Contributions of Childhood Adversity and Recent Stressors to Inflammation at Midlife: Findings from the MIDUS Study. Developmental Psychology. 2015;51(11):1630-1644. doi:10.1037/dev0000049.

29. Chanlongbutra A, Singh GK, Mueller CD. Adverse Childhood Experiences, Health Related Quality of Life, and Chronic Disease Risks in Rural Areas of the United States. *Journal of Environmental and Public Health*. 2018;2018:7151297. doi:10.1155/2018/7151297.

30. Galland L. The Gut Microbiome and the Brain. *Journal of Medicinal Food*. 2014;17(12):1261-1272. doi:10.1089/jmf.2014.7000.

31. Cenit MC, Sanz Y, Codoñer-Franch P. Influence of gut microbiota on neuropsychiatric disorders. *World Journal of Gastroenterology*. 2017;23(30):5486-5498. doi:10.3748/wjg.v23.i30.5486.

32. Mergenthaler P, Lindauer U, Dienel GA, Meisel A. Sugar for the brain: the role of glucose in physiological and pathological brain function. *Trends in neurosciences*. 2013;36(10):587-597. doi:10.1016/j.tins.2013 07.001.

33. Milton K. Hunter-gatherer diets—a different perspective. *The American Journal of Clinical Nutrition*. 200; 71(3):665-667

34. Cordain L, Miller JB, Eaton SB, Mann N, Holt S, Speth JD. Plant-animal subsistence ratios and macronutrient energy estimations in worldwide hunter-gatherer diets, *The American Journal of Clinical Nutrition*. 2000; 71(3): 682–692.

35. Prasad S, Sajja RK, Naik P, Cucullo L. Diabetes Mellitus and Blood-Brain Barrier Dysfunction: An Overview. *Journal of Pharmacovigilance*. 2014;2(2):125-. doi:10.4172/2329-6887.1000125.

36. https://www.ncld.org/the-state-of-learning-disabilities-understanding-the-1-in-5

37. http://www.nimh.nih.gov/health/statistics/prevalence/any-mental-illness-ami-among-adults.shtml

38. https://www.ncbi.nlm.nih.gov/pmc/articles/PMC1978319/

39. Semenkovich, K., Brown, M.E., Svrakic, D.M. et al. Drugs (2015) 75: 577. https://doi.org/10.1007/s40265-015-0347-4

40. Pigott H., Leventhal, A., Alter, G., & Boren, J. (2010). Efficacy and Effectiveness of Antidepressants: Current Status of Research. *Psychother Psychosom*; 79:267-279.

41. Daniel J. Cox, Boris P. Kovatchev, Linda A. Gonder-Frederick, Kent H. Summers, Anthony McCall, Kevin J. Grimm, William L. Clarke. Performance Among Adults With Type 1 and Type 2 Diabetes. *Diabetes Care*. 2005, 28 (1) 71-77; DOI: 10.2337/diacare.28.1.71

42. https://www.hopkinsmedicine.org/diabetes/diabetes_education/patient_education_material/get_off_the_blood_glucose_rollercoaster.pdf

43. Ornoy A, Wolf A, Ratzon N, et al. Neurodevelopmental outcome at early school age of children born to mothers with diabetes. *Archives of Disease in Childhood - Fetal and Neonatal Edition* 1999;81:F10-F14.

44. Timonen Markku, Laakso Mauri, Jokelainen Jari, Rajala Ulla, Meyer-Rochow V Benno, Keinänen-Kiukaanniemi Sirkka et al. Insulin resistance and depression: cross sectional study *BMJ* 2004; 330 :17

45. Linden, D. E. J., Habes, I., Johnston, S. J., Linden, S., Tatineni, R., Subramanian, L., ... Goebel, R. (2012). Real-Time Self-Regulation of Emotion Networks in Patients with Depression. *PLoS ONE*, 7(6), e38115. http://doi.org/10.1371/journal.pone.0038115

46. https://www.cdc.gov/diabetes/data/statistics/statistics-report.html

47. Rowley WR, Bezold C, Arikan Y, Byrne E, Krohe S. Diabetes 2030: Insights from Yesterday, Today, and Future Trends. *Population Health Management.* 2017;20(1):6-12. doi:10.1089/pop.2015.0181.

48. https://www.cdc.gov/media/pressrel/2010/r101022.html

49. http://www.diabetes.org/diabetes-basics/statistics/

50. https://www.cdc.gov/obesity/data/childhood.html

51. Tuso P. Prediabetes and Lifestyle Modification: Time to Prevent a Preventable Disease. *The Permanente Journal.* 2014;18(3):88-93. doi:10.7812/TPP/14-002.

52. Hernandez M, Mollo A, Marsal JR, et al. Insulin secretion in patients with latent autoimmune diabetes (LADA): half way between type 1 and type 2 diabetes: action LADA 9. *BMC Endocrine Disorders.* 2015;15:1. doi:10.1186/1472-6823-15-1.

53. De la Monte SM. Type 3 Diabetes is Sporadic Alzheimer's disease: Mini-Review. *European neuropsychopharmacology : the journal of the European College of Neuropsychopharmacology.* 2014;24(12):1954-1960. doi:10.1016/j.euroneuro.2014.06.008.

54. Bredesen DE. Metabolic profiling distinguishes three subtypes of Alzheimer's disease. *Aging (Albany NY).* 2015;7(8):595-600.

55. Partnership to Fight Chronic Disease. https://www.fightchronicdisease.org/about. Accessed July 27, 2018.

56. Wang H, Abajobir AA, Abate KH, et al. GBD 2016 Mortality Collaborators. Global, regional, and national under-5 mortality, adult mortality, age-specific mortality, and life expectancy, 1970-2016. *Lancet.* 2017;390(10100):1084-1150.

57. The US Burden of Disease Collaborators. The State of US Health, 1990-2016 Burden of Diseases, Injuries, and Risk Factors Among US States. *JAMA.* 2018;319(14):1444–1472. doi:10.1001/jama.2018.0158

58. Vighi G, Marcucci F, Sensi L, Di Cara G, Frati F. Allergy and the gastrointestinal system. Clin Exp Immunol. 2008;153 Suppl 1(Suppl 1):3-6.

59. R c t ianu N, et al. Thyroid disorders in obese patients. Does insulin resistance make a difference? *Arch Endocrinol Metab.* 2017;61(6):575-583. doi: 10.1590/2359-3997000000306.

60. Habib SL, Rojna M. Diabetes and Risk of Cancer. ISRN *Oncology.* 2013;2013:583786. doi:10.1155/2013/583786.

61. Glenn J, Stitt A. The role of advanced glycation end products in retinal ageing and disease. *Biochimica et Biophysica Acta.* 2009;1790 (10): 1109-1116.

62. Krone C, Ely J. Controlling hyperglycemia as an adjunct to cancer therapy. *Integrative Cancer Therapies.* 2005;4(1) 25–31

63. Li W, Ma Q, Liu J, et al. Hyperglycemia as a mechanism of pancreatic cancer metastasis. *Frontiers in Bioscience.* 2012;17:1761–1774, 2012

64. K. Yamasaki, Y. Hayashi, S. Okamoto, M. Osanai, and G.-H. Lee, Insulin-independent promotion of chemically induced hepatocellular tumor development in genetically diabetic mice. *Cancer Science*. 2010;101(1) 65–72.

65. Dineley KT, Jahrling JB, Denner L. Insulin resistance in Alzheimer's disease. *Neurobiol Dis*. 2014;72 Pt A:92-103.

66. Ankarcrona M, Winblad B, Monteiro C, et al. Current and future treatment of amyloid diseases. *J Intern Med*. 2016;280(2):177-202

67. Szabó M, Máté B, Csép K, Benedek T. Epigenetic Modifications Linked to T2D, the Heritability Gap, and Potential Therapeutic Targets. *Biochem Genet*. 2018 Jun 5. doi: 10.1007/s10528-018-9863-8.

68. Gomes AC, Bueno AA, de Souza RGM, Mota JF. Gut microbiota, probiotics and diabetes. *Nutrition Journal*. 2014;13:60. doi:10.1186/1475-2891-13-60.

69. Elamin M, Ruskin DN, Masino SA, Sacchetti P. Ketone-Based Metabolic Therapy: Is Increased NAD+ a Primary Mechanism?. *Front Mol Neurosci*. 2017;10:377. Published 2017 Nov 14. doi:10.3389/fnmol.2017.00377

70. Vlassara H, Striker GE. AGE restriction in diabetes mellitus: a paradigm shift. *Nat Rev Endocrinol*. 2011;7(9):526-39.

71. Veyrat-Durebex C, Reynier P, Procaccio V, et al. How Can a Ketogenic Diet Improve Motor Function? *Frontiers in Molecular Neuroscience*. 2018;11:15. doi:10.3389/fnmol.2018.00015.

72. Ruitenberg A, Kalmijn S, de Ridder MA, Redekop WK, van HF, Hofman A, et al. Prognosis of Alzheimer's disease: the Rotterdam Study. Neuroepidemiology. 2001;20:188–195.Henderson ST. High carbohydrate diets and Alzheimer's disease. Med Hypotheses. 2004;62:689–700

73. Longo VD, Panda S. Fasting, circadian rhythms, and time restricted feeding in healthy lifespan. *Cell metabolism*. 2016;23(6):1048-1059. doi:10.1016/j.cmet.2016.06.001.

74. Mattson MP. Energy intake, meal frequency, and health: a neurobiological perspective. *Annu Rev Nutr*. 2005;25:237-60.

75. Tyler WJ, Alonso M, Bramham CR, Pozzo-Miller LD. From Acquisition to Consolidation: On the Role of Brain-Derived Neurotrophic Factor Signaling in Hippocampal-Dependent Learning. *Learning & memory* (Cold Spring Harbor, NY). 2002;9

76. Cowansage KK, LeDoux JE, Monfils MH. Brain-derived neurotrophic factor: a dynamic gatekeeper of neural plasticity. *Curr Mol Pharmacol*. 2010; 3(1):12

77. Murer MG, Yan Q, Raisman-Vozari R. Brain-derived neurotrophic factor in the control human brain, and in Alzheimer's disease and Parkinson's disease. *Prog Neurobiol*. 2001; 63(1):71-124

78. Sun Q, Tang D-D, Yin E-G, et al. Diagnostic Significance of Serum Levels of Nerve Growth Factor and Brain Derived Neurotrophic Factor in Diabetic Peripheral Neuropathy. *Medical Science Monitor : International Medical Journal of Experimental and Clinical Research*. 2018;24:5943-5950. doi:10.12659/MSM.909449

79. Komulainen P, Pedersen M, Hänninen T, Bruunsgaard H, Lakka TA, Kivipelto M, Hassinen M, Rauramaa TH, Pedersen BK, Rauramaa R. BDNF is a novel marker of cognitive function in ageing women: the DR's EXTRA Study. *Neurobiol Learn Mem*. 2008; 90(4):596-603

80. Rage F, Silhol M, Binamé F, Arancibia S, Tapia-Arancibia L.Effect of aging on the expression of BDNF and TrkB isoforms in rat pituitary. *Neurobiol Aging*. 2007; 28(7):1088-98.

81. Hossein-nezhad A, Holick MF. Vitamin D for Health: A Global Perspective. Mayo Clinic proceedings *Mayo Clinic*. 2013;88(7):720-755. doi:10.1016/j.mayocp.2013.05.011.

82. Hardeland R. Neurobiology, Pathophysiology, and Treatment of Melatonin Deficiency and Dysfunction. *The Scientific World Journal*. 2012;2012:640389. doi:10.1100/2012/640389.

83. Zephy D, Ahmad J. Type 2 diabetes mellitus: Role of melatonin and oxidative stress. Diabetes & Metabolic Syndrome: *Clinical Research & Reviews*. 2015;9(2): 127-131,

84. Vincent RR, Appukuttan D, Victor DJ, Balasundaram A. Oxidative stress in chronic periodontitis patients with type II diabetes mellitus. *Eur J Dent*. 2018;12(2):225-231.

REFERENCES

85. Van Dongen HP, Maislin G, Mullington JM, Dinges DF. The cumulative cost of additional wakefulness: dose-response effects on neurobehavioral functions and sleep physiology from chronic sleep restriction and total sleep deprivation. *Sleep*. 2003; 26(2):117-26.

86. Reutrakul S, Van Cauter E. Interactions between sleep, circadian function, and glucose metabolism: implications for risk and severity of diabetes. Ann N Y *Acad Sci*. 2014.1311:151-73. doi: 10.1111/nyas.12355.

87. Sweeney EL, Jeromson S, Hamilton DL, Brooks NE, Walshe IH. Skeletal muscle insulin signaling and whole body glucose metabolism following acute sleep restriction in healthy males. *Physiological Reports*. 2017;5(23):e13498. doi:10.14814/phy2.13498

88. Giese M, Unternaehrer E, Brand S, Calabrese P, Holsboer-Trachsler E, Eckert A. The Interplay of Stress and Sleep Impacts BDNF Level *PLoS One*. 2013; 8(10): e76050

89. Hang L, Zhang HQ, Liang XY, Zhang HF, Zhang T, Liu FE. Melatonin ameliorates cognitive impairment induced by sleep deprivation in rats: role of oxidative stress, BDNF and CaMKII. *Behav Brain Res*. 2013;256:72-81. 6.

90. Lumb A. Diabetes and exercise. *Clin Med* (Lond). 2014 Dec;14(6):673-6. doi: 10.7861/clinmedicine.14-6-673.

91. Ford, E. Does Exercise Reduce Inflammation? Physical Activity and C- Reactive Protein Among U.S. Adults. *Epidemiology*. 2002(13)5: 561-568

92. Horsburgh S, Robson-Ansley P, Adams R, Smith C. Exercise and inflammation-related epigenetic modifications: focus on DNA methylation. Exerc Immunol Rev. 2015;21:26-41.

93. Saucedo Marquez CM, Vanaudenaerde B, Troosters T, Wenderoth N. High-intensity interval training evokes larger serum BDNF levels compared with intense continuous exercise. *J Appl Physiol* (1985). 2015;119(12):1363-73

94. Kerling A, et al. Exercise increases serum brain-derived neurotrophic factor in patients with major depressive disorder. *J Affect Disord*. 2017;215:152-155

95. Priya G, Kalra S. Mind–Body Interactions and Mindfulness Meditation in Diabetes. *European Endocrinology*. 2018;14(1):35-41. doi:10.17925/EE.2018.14.1.35.

96. Cahn BR, Goodman MS, Peterson CT, Maturi R, Mills PJ. Yoga, Meditation and Mind-Body Health: Increased BDNF, Cortisol Awakening Response, and Altered Inflammatory Marker Expression after a 3-Month Yoga and Meditation Retreat. *Front Hum Neurosci*. 2017;11:315. Published 2017 Jun 26. doi:10.3389/fnhum.2017.00315

97. Hossein-nezhad A, Holick MF. Vitamin D for Health: A Global Perspective. *Mayo Clinic proceedings Mayo Clinic*. 2013;88(7):720-755. doi:10.1016/j.mayocp.2013.05.011.

98. Hoogendijk WJG, Lips P, Dik MG, Deeg DJH, Beekman ATF, Penninx BWJH. Depression Is Associated With Decreased 25-Hydroxyvitamin D and Increased Parathyroid Hormone Levels in Older Adults. *Arch Gen Psychiatry*. 2008;65(5):508–512. doi:10.1001/archpsyc.65.5.508

99. Tabatabaei-Malazy O, Salari P, Khashayar P, Larijani B. New horizons in treatment of osteoporosis. *DARU Journal of Pharmaceutical Sciences*. 2017;25:2. doi:10.1186/s40199-017-0167-z.

100. Colaris MJL, van der Hulst RR, Tervaert JWC. Vitamin D deficiency as a risk factor for the development of autoantibodies in patients with ASIA and silicone breast implants: a cohort study and review of the literature. *Clinical Rheumatology*. 2017;36(5):981-993. doi:10.1007/s10067-017-3589-6.

101. Cantorna MT, Snyder L, Lin Y-D, Yang L. Vitamin D and 1,25(OH)2D Regulation of T cells. *Nutrients*. 2015;7(4):3011-3021. doi:10.3390/nu7043011.

102. Fondjo LA, Sakyi SA, Owiredu WKBA, et al. Evaluating Vitamin D Status in Pre- and Postmenopausal Type 2 Diabetics and Its Association with Glucose Homeostasis. *BioMed Research International*. 2018;2018:9369282. doi:10.1155/2018/9369282

103. Hossein-nezhad A, Holick MF. Vitamin D for Health: A Global Perspective. *Mayo Clinic proceedings Mayo Clinic*. 2013;88(7):720-755. doi:10.1016/j.mayocp.2013.05.011.

104. Hardeland R. Neurobiology, Pathophysiology, and Treatment of Melatonin Deficiency and Dysfunction. *The Scientific World Journal*. 2012;2012:640389. doi:10.1100/2012/640389.

105. Zephy D, Ahmad J. Type 2 diabetes mellitus: Role of melatonin and oxidative stress. *Diabetes & Metabolic Syndrome: Clinical Research & Reviews.* 2015; 9(2):127-131.

106. Gomes AC, Bueno AA, de Souza RGM, Mota JF. Gut microbiota, probiotics and diabetes. *Nutrition Journal.* 2014;13:60. doi:10.1186/1475-2891-13-60.

107. Lee W, Song K, Koh E, Won J, KimH, Park H, Kim M, Kim S, Lee K, Park J. -Lipoic acid increases insulin sensitivity by activating AMPK in skeletal muscle, *Biochemical and Biophysical Research Communications.* 2005; 332(3):885-891,

108. Rochette L, Ghibu S, Muresan A, Vergely C. Alpha-lipoic acid: molecular mechanisms and therapeutic potential in diabetes. *Canadian Journal of Physiology and Pharmacology.* 2015;92:1021-27.

109. Song Y, Ridker PM, Manson JE, Cook NR, Buring JE, Liu S. Magnesium intake, C-reactive protein, and the prevalence of metabolic syndrome in middle-aged and older U.S. women. *Diabetes Care.* 2005; 28(6):1438-44.

110. 110.Ma J., Folsom A.R., Melnick S.L., Eckfeldt J.H., Sharrett A.R., Nabulsi A.A., Hutchinson R.G., Metcalf P.A. Associations of serum and dietary magnesium with cardiovascular disease, hypertension, diabetes, insulin, and carotid arterial wall thickness: The ARIC study. Atherosclerosis Risk in Communities Study. *J. Clin. Epidemiol.* 1995;48:927–940.

111. Gröber U, Schmidt J, Kisters K. Magnesium in Prevention and Therapy. *Nutrients.* 2015;7(9):8199-8226. doi:10.3390/nu7095388

ABOUT THE AUTHOR

Dr Ben Galyardt, D.C., Founder and CEO of F8 Well Centers, and The Galyardt Method is a leading expert and speaker in Functional Medicine, Neurofeedback and Brain Regeneration. Specializing in blood sugar and brain rejuvenation, Dr Galyardt has helped thousands of people return to optimal health by digging deep and finding the root cause of chronic health issues.

Dr. Galyardt grew up in an active family that stressed the importance of nutrition and a healthy lifestyle so a major illness was not something they worried about. That all changed his junior year of High School while playing a football game his mom collapsed and had to be carried to the emergency room. The following months were filled with doctor visits and tests. She was diagnosed with Multiple Sclerosis (MS) – an unpredictable, often disabling autoimmune disease of the central nervous system that disrupts the flow of information within the brain and between the brain and body.

Conforming to the traditional medical route to treat the disease, Mrs. Galyardt was prescribed every drug available with little to no success. She resigned herself to the aid of a cane to walk and an electric cart for the grocery store.

Eventually she realized she needed something more than medication. Looking for other alternatives to treat her disease, Dr. Galyardt's mother decided to see a Functional Medicine doctor. It changed her life. She became empowered to take an active role in learning about her body and its ability to heal itself. Because of the Functional Medicine methods, the last MRI results showed zero plaque left on the spine or brain. The Neurologist was dumbfounded and could not comprehend how her body had stopped the damage, and reversed the scarred areas.

She is now able to do granny bootcamp, shop, fish, hike and take care of her 7 grandchildren, all done without the mainstream medications prescribed for MS.

Dr Ben was hooked on learning more about Functional Medicine which incorporates the latest in genetic science, systems biology, as well as an understanding of how environmental and lifestyle factors influence the emergence and progression of disease. He has spent the rest of his life learning these methods from the top name doctors across the country. He was an expert in Functional Medicine before it was even called Functional Medicine.

When his wife was also diagnosed with Lyme and autoimmune to the brain despite a healthy diet and lifestyle he knew there had to be more to health than just eating "healthy" food. As he studied how to help her recover he started learning more about how blood sugar affects all systems in the body and how blood sugar imbalances, with regular spikes and crashes, lead to inflammation and improper stimulation of the immune system.

He began testing her and more of his patients' blood sugar to see what he would find and sure enough the more variability there was in a patients' blood sugar the more chronic disease they would have. He now uses blood sugar monitoring as a staple in patient care.

Dr. Galyardt's Board Certifications, Degrees and Training include:

- Board Certified in Integrative Medicine

- Certified Neurofeedback Practitioner

- International College Applied Kinesiology (AK)

- Neuro-Emotional Technique (NET) Certification

- Trigenics Practitioner

- Certified by the American Functional Institute in Functional Neurology

- Advanced Muscle Integration Technique (AMIT)

- Autonomic Response Testing (ART) by Dr. Dietrich Klinghardt

- Bachelors from Syracuse University in Health and Exercise Science

- Graduated from Parker College of Chiropractic in Dallas, Texas

- CEO and Founder of F8 Well Centers in Fort Collins Colorado and Tennessee

He works with patients in his Colorado office as well as training and mentoring the doctors that run F8 Well Centers' offices across the country. When not at the office he enjoys hiking, fishing, hunting and paddle boarding with his wife and 4 boys.

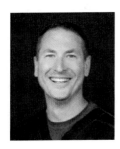

Dr. Ben Galyardt

Owner of F8 Well Centers &
Pioneer of the Galyardt Method

Made in the USA
Middletown, DE
01 April 2023

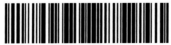

28089657R00088